How To Ma
Clothes & Be Stylish For A Lifetime

2nd SKIN

Sarah Tinks Cross

Copyright © 2024 Sarah Cross

All rights reserved.

No part of this book may be reproduced, or stored in a retrieval system, or transmitted in any form or by any means, electronic, mechanical, photocopying, recording, or otherwise, without express written permission of the copyright holder.

Note that the advice and methods in this book are not guaranteed success. Success depends on active participation. This book is sold with the understanding that the author is not held responsible for outcomes resulting from actioning the advice herein.

The stories, case studies, and scenarios, portrayed in this book are based on real life events and results. Names and some details have been changed to respect the privacy of clients.

ISBN: 9798339524434

Cover design by: Sarah Cross

*This book is dedicated to Liberty, Leo, Adrian and Henry.
Every day you fill my world with endless love and
make me a better person.
Thank you.*

*&
In loving memory of
Elizabeth Pauline Taylor.*

CONTENTS

Copyright
Dedication
Introduction   1
1. You Laid Bare   15
2. Clothes Unpicked   75
3. Style Formulas   126
4. Daily Dress Code   149
5. Wardrobe Therapy - Part 1   176
6. Wardrobe Therapy - Part 2   210
7. Evolving Your UPS   235
8. Finishing Touches   286
9. The Wardrobe Evolution Cycle   313
10. Not The End   318
Glossary   321
Resources   327
Acknowledgements   329
About the Author   332

Introduction

"Hi, if I knew you were coming, I would have worn..."

―――――――― • ――――――――

Confessions of getting dressed, or more to the point, the exhausting cycle of finding something to wear, is a subject of discussion I find myself having most days. It's not a conversation I instigate, though; it comes when I am complimented on my outfit, and the person I am talking to realises I am a personal stylist.

That's when the floodgates open:

> "I used to love clothes when I was younger."
> "My clothes are comfortable, so style doesn't matter."
> "Nothing fits me because my body is an unusual shape."
> "When I lose some weight, I'll start thinking about clothes again."
> "I don't have the time or money since the family have taken priority."
> "I'm not happy with my figure, so I'm not investing in clothes right now."

The conversation continues, interspersed with some of my own confessions:

> "I know what you mean; I have no idea at what age my size started fluctuating, both in size labels and on the scales..."
> "I used to love shopping; it was a day out. I couldn't walk in those heels now."
> "The weights creeping back on... Thank goodness for stretch..."

And then, I'll throw in a conversation stopper:

> "You shouldn't have to justify what you choose to wear."

This is the absolute truth, but... we are all battling our frustrations when choosing what to wear.

Here are some all-too-common examples:

"I would love to wear nice clothes, but I don't know where to start."

"My body has changed shape, and my usual clothes don't feel right anymore."

"When I tried wearing something different, I received comments."

"Nothing fits my body, and I don't know what suits me anyway."

"I stare at my wardrobe, and my heart sinks; I have nothing to wear."

What I've discovered is that these 'truths' and 'frustrations' come primarily from an intrinsic lack of confidence in knowing what to own and wear to create our unique, stylish look.

So, here's the good news: It *is* possible to open your wardrobe door and feel your mood elevate, no matter what is happening in your life. I know that sounds way out of reach right now, but I promise, by the end of this book, you will have acquired all the tools you need to make more considered and determined choices. Once you make those, everything you choose to wear will reflect exactly who you are and not who you think you should be.

2nd SKIN will teach you the principles and steps required to continually evolve a collection of clothes that make you feel good, look your best, and are appropriate to your lifestyle, whatever age or stage you are at. The concepts I introduce will debunk the myths and cast aside the worn-out clichés whilst avoiding generic advice. Plus, we will be diving deep into unchartered territory.

2nd SKIN will empower you to dress with more definition, confidence, and ease. What's more, these steps will also transform your existing wardrobe, moving it away from the exhausting cycle of having to find something to wear and presenting instead a choice of ready-to-wear outfits for any occasion—all right there at your fingertips.

It's been three decades since I started my professional love affair with clothes, having graduated (rather proudly) in 1994 with my BA(Hons) Degree in Fashion. My career path commenced working as a junior pattern cutter before, over the years, working my way up to become one of the senior designers in London fashion houses. On-the-job experience at the sharp end of fashion and garment design taught me so much about what goes into the mix to create the perfect item of clothing, ranging from its fabric to its cut, fit and shape.

Later in my career, I took the position of lead Lecturer of Fashion & Clothing, which coincided with a time when more and more women began asking for my help with their style, confidence, and daily dressing. To meet their needs and offer as many solutions as I could, I added Personal Colour Analysis to my repertoire and was subsequently rewarded with the 'Best Image Consultant Newcomer 2013' award.

Fast forward to 2019, when I was shocked to be recognised for my innovation in Sustainable Wardrobe Editing. I had been altering garments, and sourcing high-quality pre-loved clothing at budget-conscious prices for years, so to be recognised in this way for something that I loved was incredibly humbling. As an even greater bonus, the prize for this recognition came in the form of funding, which spurred me on to set up my own company, MYVOS®, aka My Very Own Stylist – Personal Styling & Wardrobe Editing Services.

One of the most important lessons I have learnt is that someone telling you what to wear will not make you stylish. An article in a magazine, a blog, a Google search, or a stand-alone 3-hour session with a personal shopper won't fulfil the role either. Whilst the latter is undoubtedly an enjoyable experience, each of these are only temporary fixes which, though a starting point, form only a small part of the investment you are about to make in finding, improving and loving your own unique style.

If you are seeking a genuine, eternal, effortless style that ultimately uses what you wear to elevate your mood whilst bringing joy, confidence, and well-being to your life every day, we need to delve into the nooks of how your visual communication—aka Personal Style—is created.

But what is Personal Style?

Personal Style starts with your body, closely followed by your existing clothes collection. These two are then matched to align with your daily lifestyle. What is important to remember here is that all three elements – body, clothes and lifestyle - are unique to you and will change over time. One size, one look, and one style do not fit forever, so the chapters in this book will guide you through how to evolve your clothes at the same pace as your body and lifestyle. Through 2nd SKIN, you will gain the necessary knowledge to prepare for and follow a Five-Step-Cycle which allows your clothes to meet you exactly where you're at – regardless of age, money, body type and lifestyle.

When my client, Becky, aged 44, a full-time business analyst and mother to 6-year-old Millie, cited budget and time as the primary reasons preventing her from managing her clothes and dressing well, I knew this wasn't the whole truth. But I also realised that the only way I could shift Becky's mindset and give her the confidence boost she needed was to persuade her to let me into her wardrobe for a second time. I had briefly worked with Becky before on a couple of specific outfit combinations, so I had an idea of how she felt about clothes.

Since this previous occasion, Becky's body shape had adjusted a little, and she was up a dress size on her bottom half. Her daughter's needs had also changed – she'd started school - and Becky's work environment was significantly different; she regularly worked from home as opposed to a more formal office environment. The change in routine at home and work meant that Becky's daily dressing style had become more casual, and she no longer bothered with footwear or coats. Equally, she stopped considering finishing touches such as bags, accessories, and make-up, although she never missed the monthly hair appointments she'd always loved.

Becky had understandably defaulted into a 'make do' method of dressing that took no account of her personal style or, indeed, dressing for her lifestyle. Although she recognised her clothes were not making her feel good or doing any favours for her figure, she didn't know what her style was or what clothes to buy. So, it wasn't money or time preventing her from dressing well; Becky's truth was rooted in deeper self-esteem issues, body image, and change.

In the immortal words of Mr Dior, who knows a bit about dressing stylishly…

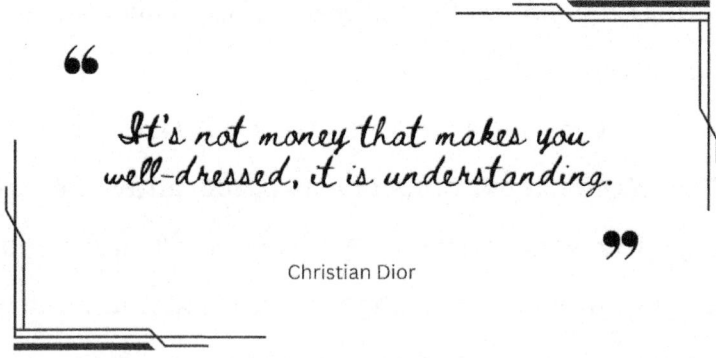

> *It's not money that makes you well-dressed, it is understanding.*
>
> Christian Dior

Becky is not the only client who has cited time as an issue; however, if you think about it, getting dressed doesn't actually take that long. What eats into our precious hours are the years we spend buying yet another fashion faux pas, going through the returns process, starting the garment search again, deciphering what suits us and so on. When I talk about 'managing your wardrobe', this time relates primarily to acquiring the garments in the first instance. If you have a wardrobe bursting with fashion faux pas clothing that didn't get returned, subpar choices made in a rush, clothes that no longer fit, or items that don't align with your current daily life – then you're not managing your wardrobe, it is managing you and taking up far too much of your time.

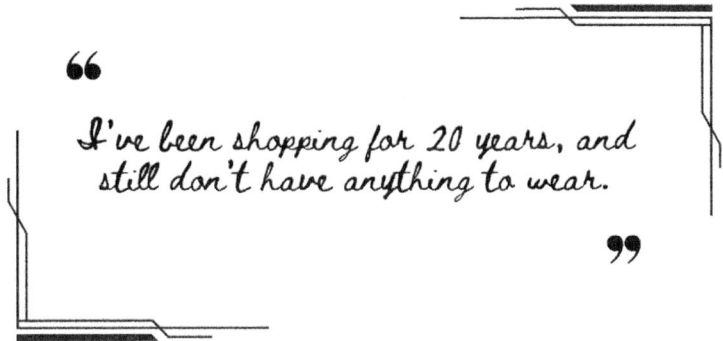

> I've been shopping for 20 years, and still don't have anything to wear.

I want to add an important caveat at this stage. Though I've talked about 2nd SKIN and my Five-Step-Cycle, you won't find this revealed in full until the penultimate chapter, which may feel odd, but bear with me; I have a good reason. You see, in order for you to gain the most from 2nd SKIN and my Five-Step-Cycle, you have to have a degree of knowledge first. It is not about providing you with a quick fix or something that you can do once and never worry about your wardrobe again; it is a practical method which works with you and your wardrobe as you both continue to evolve. With this method, you can learn how to implement my guidance and become stylish forever, which means getting off that shopping, returns, shopping cycle for good.

And to make it even easier, I've shared stories and scenarios along the way, just like Becky's. These stories are from real clients whose lives you can relate to; I've just changed their names to protect their privacy.

Before I close out this section, the one question we need to answer, the one concept we need to understand, is this though: What actually *is* style? Because this is the key to everything you are about to learn. So, let's find out.

What is Style?

In its simplest terms, Style relates to how we dress and is more commonly referred to as our 'Personal Style' when we talk about our clothing.

There are many variable definitions, such as *'Style is a feeling, an expression, a fashion trend, an outer armour, our identity, an extension of personality, a cover-up…'* However, the truth is that we all interpret Style and what it means to us differently.

You get dressed every day; we all do. It's a legal requirement if you want to leave the privacy of your home and a necessity if you want to stay warm in the colder months.

What you wear each day is a representation of you, visually and emotionally - and it's the emotional aspect of this that gets tricky. Visual is easy; that's the bit you see and read about, the abundance of Style advice in every magazine, advert, social media post, etc. But the emotional element is harder to execute and often, this is the missing element when we lose our way with Style. Often, we mistake this as a symptom of getting older, but that isn't the case. We *can* reclaim our emotional Style, and it is important to do so because Style, Dressing, Clothing or even Fashion, whatever you choose to call it, conclusively forms a key aspect of the human experience, and I, for one, want us to enjoy the human experience before we really do get taken over by AI, Bots and Aliens.

This book will help you find your Unique Personal Style (UPS), which will ultimately evolve to benefit you and your lifestyle and, **most importantly, elevate your well-being.**

Before we move on, I'd like you to take a moment and ask yourself these questions:

1. Are you 100% happy with your current collection of clothes?

2. Do you always know what clothes suit you?
3. Want to learn how to buy well? (fashion faux pas are a waste of money)
4. Do your clothes make you feel good and look the best you can?
5. Would you like to use the way you dress to bring you joy, increase your confidence, and elevate your well-being?

Don't worry about how you answered these for now. You can find, check or improve your answers as we go along because this is not just a book about clothes – it's a book that will help you **craft a visual narrative that aligns with who you are.**

Whether you feel overwhelmed by choices, unsure of what suits you, or stuck in a style rut, 2nd SKIN is your guide to sartorial self-discovery. There are no dictated trends; instead, it explores the art of personal style, helping you unearth what makes you feel comfortable, confident, and unapologetically you.

Professor *Carolyn Mair*, author of *The Psychology of Fashion*, sums it up perfectly:

INTRODUCTION | 13

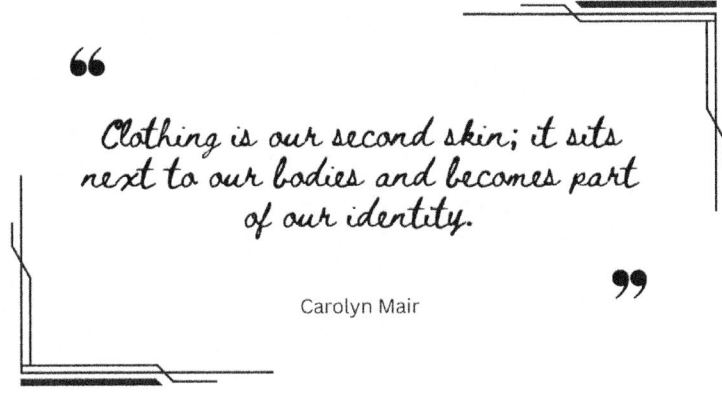

> Clothing is our second skin; it sits next to our bodies and becomes part of our identity.
>
> Carolyn Mair

So, my final question is this: Are you ready for an extraordinary expedition into the depths of Personal Style?

I hope so because together, we will shatter limitations and unlock the secrets to creating a style that truly reflects who you are. We will also navigate the complexities of body image while touching on the obstacles of self-esteem to emerge proudly with a newfound appreciation for the transformative power of clothing.

Let the journey begin!

The imagery and photographs used in this book are women ranging in size from UK6-UK22, height 5'-5'11",
Weight – well women don't give that away.
Shape – human, and outfits are their own.

Photos can be viewed at www.myvos.co.uk/2nd-skin

14 | 2ND SKIN

or by scanning the following QR Code

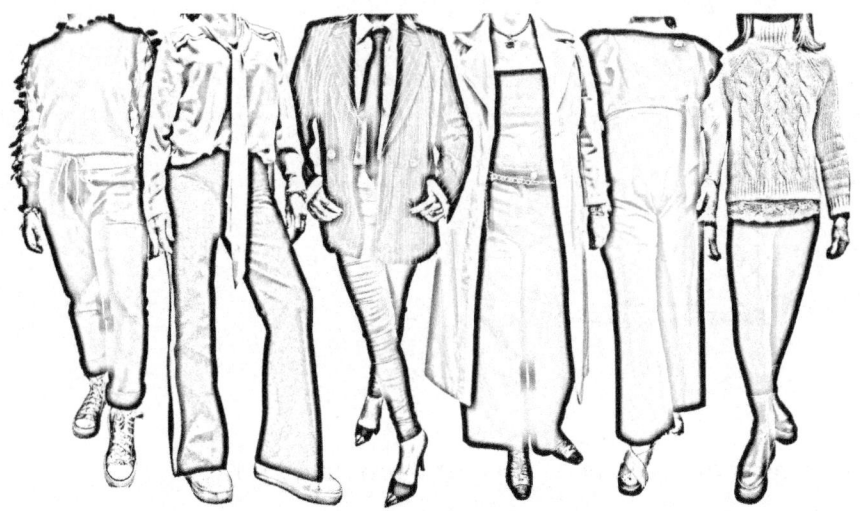

5'0" Size08 | 5'6" Size12 | 5'2" Size14 | 5'5" Size14 | 5'10" Size18 | 5'2"Size06

1. You Laid Bare

―――――•―――――

Without your body, there is nothing to clothe.

Think about that for a moment. In order to write a book about your wardrobe, we are going to have to talk - even if you're hiding behind the cushions for this entire chapter - about YOUR BODY.

Here's a question: Are you ready to embrace the beauty of your body and the quirks of ageing? Because hands up, how many times have you looked in the mirror and disliked your reflection, or worse, avoided looking in the mirror altogether?

Yep, me too, yet here's the thing: Your body and the passage of time are anything but negative. The problem isn't with our bodies; it's with the constant re-conditioning we go through to maintain a positive outlook—and this is why we all need a wardrobe edit—so that we can learn how to clothe our bodies in a way that makes us effortlessly positive (and come out from behind the cushions!).

Before we get there, though, I'd like to share a whimsical gem of humour:

The Geography of a Woman as she ages:

Age 18-25: A woman is like Africa - Half discovered, half wild, fertile, and naturally beautiful.

Age 26-33: A woman is like Europe – Well-developed and open to trade, especially to someone of real value.

Age 34-41: A woman is like Spain - Very hot, relaxed, and convinced of her own beauty.

Age 42-50: A woman is like Greece - Gently ageing but still a warm and inviting place to visit.

Age 51-60: A woman is like Great Britain - Has a glorious and all-conquering past.

Age 61-70: A woman is like Canada - Self-preserving, but open to meeting new people.

After 70: A woman is like Tibet - Wildly beautiful, with a mysterious past, the wisdom of age, an adventurous spirit, and a thirst for spiritual knowledge.

The Geography of a Male as he ages:

Age 1-100: A man is like North Korea & Russia. Ruled by a pair of nuts!

It is not scientifically accurate by any stretch of the imagination, but it is a great witty ditty and marvellous introduction to thinking positively about maturing bodies. Thank you, *@Lancelot_rebirth,* for sharing these words on your Instagram reel.

In this first chapter, we will examine your style history, discuss how our bodies change as we age, and delve into matters of the mind. The purpose of this is to help you understand where you are in your style journey and find the most logical starting point.

To begin then, I need to introduce you to the 'style tribe'.

1.1 The Style Tribe

A Tribe can be referenced as a group of people who live and work together in a shared geographical area and have a common culture, dialect, and religion. They also have a strong sense of unity, and a chief (usually) heads the Tribe.

So, what does a Tribe have to do with Style?

The answer lies in putting the two words together: style and tribe. You may not have heard of them, but 'style tribes' are simply communities of people who share the same clothes style – and they do exist. Without knowing, you will almost certainly have belonged to various 'style tribes' instigated and led by a 'chief' who 'decides' what its tribe members wear. Think about school, for example. You would have been given a uniform code in which you had little to no input; the school 'chiefs' decided what you wore every day. It's the same when you were first born and then began growing up; your tribe would have formed around what your parents or guardians chose, and then in later years, fashion trends dictated by celebrities, perhaps. These are all 'style tribes'.

By revisiting *your* **style tribes**, you can recall what you used to wear, building a history of your own personal style. This is important because, as I've indicated from the start, this book is all about *you* and *your* choice of clothing, so even though there is merit in discussing the history of fashion, that serves primarily as an interest piece rather than a foundation on which to grow your own sense of style. Hence, looking back in this way is, in my experience, the best way to move forward.

Let's consider this in a bit more depth:

- When you were born, your dressing needs were taken care of by parents, guardians and carers – in other words, the 'chiefs' in a newborn's life.
- At school, a code of uniform would have been provided by the 'school chiefs'.
- As you got older, your influences would have come from those outside of your immediate world, such as celebrities or people you admired. It's all about mirroring what you love and striving to fit in— becoming part of *their* tribe.
- In the workplace, there might be a policy on workwear – maybe even a uniform – think sectors such as the emergency services, carers, and fast-food workers. It is my guess that there are more workplaces with workwear policies than those that haven't. Here, you are fitting into the workplace tribe – again dictated to by 'chiefs' from your place of employment.

- Style tribes can also be born from the expectations of a predecessor or simply your environment (think beachwear).

If you take a moment to consider, you'll realise that there has been a huge variation in what led you away from the safety of childhood dressing, where you made little to no decisions, to following your chosen tribe - or even fending for yourself and becoming a trendsetter! It's not even a conscious concept – we just instinctively get dressed.

In the early 1990s, **style tribes** changed considerably when the *'luxury'* of *'fast fashion'* emerged. A term first used in a New York Times article, *'fast fashion',* was used to explain clothing brand Zara's goal of using manufacturing processes which enabled them to take a garment from design through production and into their retail outlets within fifteen days.

This speed of mass garment production was, at the time, unheard of. Previously, clothing had been scarcer and more expensive, leading to many of the older generations making their own clothing because it was cheaper to buy the material and quicker than waiting for (new season) fashions to appear in the shops. Those who weren't making their clothes would save until they could afford to buy what they wanted or wait for the once-a-season sale. Back then, clothing was more than something to cover our bodies; it was an indicator of class and status, meaning that your wealth and skills directly contributed to which **style tribe** you were able to belong to.

Fast fashion changed all that. It brought accessibility, freedom of choice, and affordability to clothing—never had we been presented with so many attainable options. However, its impact on the demise of modern-day dress codes cannot be ignored. Where formal wear and Sunday best were regular staples, now they are consigned to occasions such as weddings, funerals, milestone celebrations, and ceremonies.

(**Note** – these events will have a **style tribe** chief, too. Often, the person organisation or company hosting the event will set the dress code, and an expectation is placed on the guests to adhere – and don't we love it if someone doesn't adhere? What an opportunity to analyse and scrutinise the human who falls a whisker short of being well-dressed at such prestigious affairs).

One of the most recognisable **style tribes** comes from music—think punks, goths, hippies, ravers, and the like. Anthropologist Ted Polhemus analyses Style Tribes in several of his books and concludes they are not (as perhaps initially thought) limited only to Gen Z (those born between 1997 and

2012); in fact, they are quite the opposite. It has even been suggested that Ted Polhemus was the first to coin the phrase, 'style tribe'.

Style Tribe - Summary

- The availability of *fast fashion*, lower price tags, and relaxed social boundaries have opened the floodgates to an overwhelming amount of clothing choices.
- The result for the consumer is wardrobe confusion and endless 'what-to-wear dilemmas'.
- What's more, the speed of this clothing revolution has been so swift that (most) predecessor **'style tribes'** are now outdated and no longer align with current culture.
- Today, defining your boundaries and creating your own **style tribe** rules is like renovating a period property. It's all about balancing your 'stylish' past, incorporating 'mod cons' and making it seamlessly cohesive to complete your overall look.

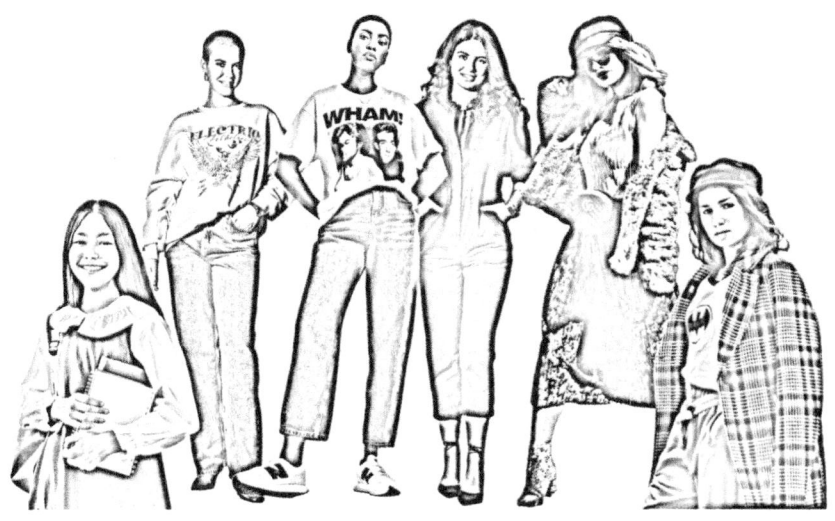

Remember Your First Style?

Suggested Actions:

In preparation for moving forward to manage your current wardrobe, think about your ideal personal style and how you would like to be seen. Ask yourself:

1. Do you want to be part of a **style tribe** and follow a set style?
2. Are you more of a chief who does your own thing, like a trendsetter?
3. How do you feel about a (repetitive) restricted look that reduces decision-making?
4. Or are you striving to always look good, feel confident, and be comfy?

24 | 2ND SKIN

1.2 Style History & Your Fashionable Future

Uniforms are undoubtedly on the demise in places where we have a certain freedom of choice (think corporate). A decrease in the use of terms such as 'white-collar workers' and 'blue-collar workers' has met with the introduction of 'dress-down Friday' and, more recently, the insurgence of loungewear - which is basically a posh version of pyjamas.

Loungewear became popular during the 2020 COVID-19 pandemic and has retained its appeal, particularly given the increase in those who have continued to work from home. Predominantly worn around the house, it is not nightwear as such and is therefore considered acceptable to casual visitors. Some also believe it appropriate to wear outside of the house when running errands, for example.

Similarly, other features that would have distinguished us from previously recognised **style tribes,** such as tattoos, hair colours in rainbow shades, facial hair and facial piercing, are no longer 'discouraged' and are trends increasingly seen in the office space that was previously occupied by the white-collar **style tribes** (in some workplaces, these 'distinguishing' features were formerly forbidden).

Senior industry CEOs have gone on to create an *'entitlement dress code'*, which permits wearing T-shirts and trainers in boardroom meetings. However, there are still limits. An *'entitlement dresser'* should be *'well-groomed with a calculated stylish yet casual look'*, not a *'rushed, nothing to wear, sloppy 'loungewear' casual'* look.

These are a few of my many observations surrounding the changing and continuously evolving way that society displays its clothing and style acceptance – and if we go deeper, we can see that it's not just limited to workplace wear either.

The off-duty dress code differs greatly from what it was even thirty years ago, and there is a definite reduction in its formality. If you look back at old photos of previous generations from the 1950s through to the 1980s, everyone looks like they are dressed pretty much in the same style. Arguably, clothing choices could be considered almost like a uniform with very little injection of personal style.

Change can be unnerving, or it can be viewed as an opportunity to take control of your own style chief. If you're good at it, you may even instigate a new **style tribe** (steady on!), which brings me back to the purpose of this chapter and a statement that I genuinely believe is key:

> *The more you know about yourself and what you want to represent, the easier it is to make confident, style choices going forward.*

Style History – Summary

- The reduction of rules and the onus of what to wear being put directly onto us, whilst refreshing personal freedom for some, can be another added life stress for others, and both feelings are equally important.
- Regardless, though, more than ever, it is our responsibility to get what we wear 'right' for our well-being.
- Confusing messages are filtering down from the world's top leaders who can often be seen wearing casual on repeat – does that mean we should do the same?
- In addition, excessive clothing options are causing disconcerting buying habits – we can have a wardrobe that's fit to burst and still feel as if we have nothing to wear.

- These current societal trends make it all the more confusing when it comes to defining clothing boundaries and knowing what on earth to wear.

Suggested Actions:

To make sense of this mind-boggling abundance of style freedom and continue focusing on you, let's reflect on your past iconic style moments with some simple, memory-stirring questions. Questions that will generate a response like, "*Ooooh, I remember!*" and then cause either joy or embarrassment, depending upon your recollection.

> *Full disclosure:* As a teenager, I loved Boy George – now there's a memory. On one occasion, I remember braiding my hair into skinny plaits intertwined with ribbons and a few beads that I somehow managed to sew into the ends of my messy braids. The final touch, just before going to my local disco, was the addition of a hat. Though that may sound closer to what would today be considered fancy dress, I can assure you it wasn't. It was simply me loving the look of my **style tribe** and being proud to be a fan, so trust me; there are absolutely no judgements here!

Also, just because we're revisiting your past sartorial choices, that doesn't mean they will form your new capsule collection

—so don't panic. It's part of the deep-dive process of using your personal style history to understand what made you feel good and emotional in the past. This helps to discover where you stand today and how to dress tomorrow.

When answering these questions, think about your biggest influences and craziest times, although there's no need to answer a question if nothing springs to mind. A good way of going about this is remembering funny, happy moments around what you used to wear. You may want to refer to someone else in your life at that time, too. Perhaps someone you vividly remember because of what they wore, maybe a friend or relative, or even a neighbour. There are no right or wrong answers here; just let the memories and inspiration flow.

As a teenager:
1. Who or what influenced the way you dressed? Pop stars, music genres, actors, shops, magazines, peers, older siblings, a passionate pastime…
2. How did you obtain most of your clothes? Hand-me-downs bought all your own clothes, parents/guardians decided, clothes were not important enough to care about…
3. What memories do you have of a favourite garment or memorable outfit? Is it linked to a place, person, or

pastime, or is there a story attached…

Moving onto to your 20s & 30s:
1. How do you recall your style evolving from a minor to an adult?
2. What fashion trends and personal lifestyle changes were happening at that time?
3. Did you have any icons or key people that influenced your wardrobe choices?

Entering your 40s:
1. Have/did you gravitate towards a specific style or way of dressing that is/was more habit than choice? If yes, how would you describe your habitual 40s wardrobe?
2. What is/was your most significant wardrobe difference from your 20s to 40s?
3. Were/are you losing your identity or gaining confidence? How do you know?
4. Do you have items in your wardrobe that are 15+ years old? If yes, what pieces are they?

For the fabulous people in your 50s (I am one of you):
1. How do you describe your current style?
2. Have you discovered any fashion secrets or favourite pieces that make you feel confident and gorgeous that you wouldn't have considered wearing before?
3. What are the oldest items of clothing that you still

wear?

60 is the new 40

Ask yourself the same questions as entering your 40s, adding on two decades.

Compare your answers and see if any are the same.

70 is the new 50

You know what to do: Answer the 50s questions, adding two or more decades, and again compare your answers. Also, are you feeling like Tibet from our earlier 'witty ditty'? *"Wildly beautiful, with a mysterious past, the wisdom of age, an adventurous spirit, and a thirst for spiritual knowledge."*

I hope you enjoyed reflecting on your style memories and sharing any funny and fond stories. Save your answers for later; they will be useful as you grow and build knowledge of your future wardrobe.

Note Writing Space

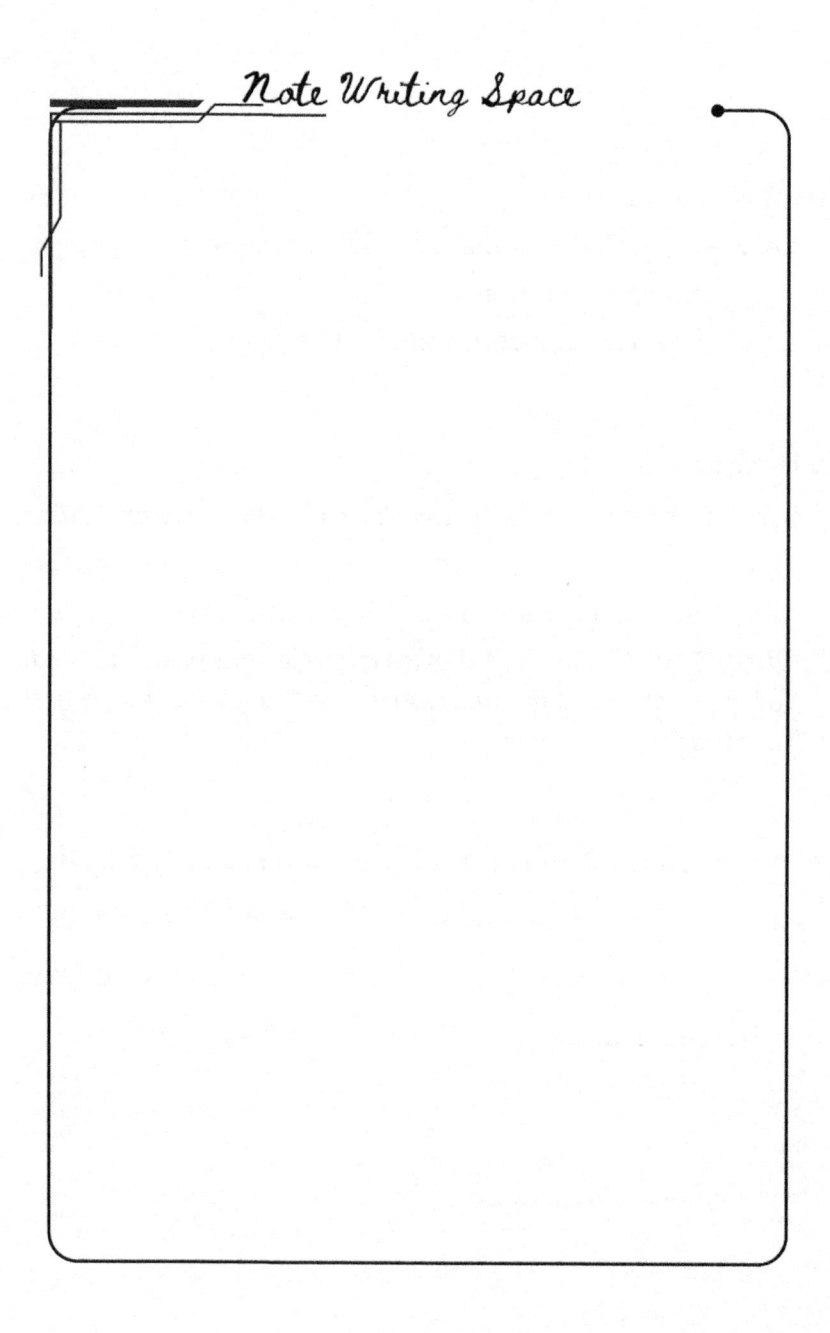

1.3 Age & Dressing

If you think about it, most things in life improve with age. Gardens mature, fine wines develop in texture and flavour, and of course, we benefit from the wisdom we gain daily.

When it comes to wisdom, research doesn't reference age explicitly; however, it is suggested that wisdom increases steadily from the ages of 13 to 25 before remaining stable (relatively speaking) up to the age of 75. Taking this literally, did your greatest experience of dress sense peak at 25?

If you refer back to your earlier answers, I'm guessing not; plus, we also need to take into account any visual signs of ageing along with the natural changes to our body shape over the years. This reinforces my belief that it is not good to have an ageing wardrobe and why our clothing collection should not be unattended for too long. If our choices, wisdom, and bodies have changed, then what we wear must change, too, and it is this knowledge we use and draw on because they (wisdom and shape changes) form the fundamental elements of creating and retaining a stylish collection of clothes.

In the book, 'BOOM! A Baby Boomer Memoir, 1947-2022', another masterpiece by anthropologist Ted Polhemus, the question of whether age is a critical boundary marker is raised. When I shared the first draft introduction of this book with Ted, he asked me, *"Does being 40+ actually make a real difference?"*. Ted certainly isn't convinced age makes any difference to dressing stylishly, and I concur. Here's why.

I have observed, witnessed, and listened to hundreds of women as they share how they feel about their clothes, usually at a time when I'm knee-deep in their wardrobes, checking every item piece by piece. During my work, I have come to realise that the age of 40 is the approximate tipping point for a woman, a time when she begins to feel in need of guidance around her clothing choices.

This need for guidance arises for many reasons; typically, she either doubts her ability and confidence in what to wear, or she's become overwhelmed by the sheer volume of clothing she already owns. Often, women at this life stage will have made additional purchases in a bid to find the answer, yet these purchases are not exciting to them, nor is her existing wardrobe of over-worn garments. Put simply, she has too many clothes, too much choice – her wardrobe is overgrown. This is a pattern I see a lot.

Going back to our ageing and mature garden for a moment, if it is not consistently maintained, if shrubs are not pruned, if plants are not treated for insect infestation, if new species of plant are introduced without consideration of the existing foliage, if the grass is not cut, if the flowers are not watered, if the weeds are not removed … you get the idea … the entire garden becomes so overgrown that it is no longer recognised as the beautiful landscape it once was. In my experience, exactly the same thing happens with our wardrobe and what's more, it can take less than a decade for the view that we peruse every day when deciding what to wear, to become unrecognisable. If a wardrobe remains untouched for more than two decades, then it is inevitably full of mature pieces, items that have seen better days, impulse buys and quick-fix purchases that simply clog up the decision-making process.

This definition is what I fondly call an *ageing wardrobe* and hands up, we've probably all been (or still are!) there. And that's fine, that's normal. If your wardrobe *doesn't* look like this, then arguably, you don't need to read this book, but if your wardrobe *does* look like this, take heart in the fact that you are not alone, ageing wardrobes are everywhere and it's okay to live with one. I promise. The goal of this book, though, is to help you recognise what does and doesn't work within what you already own and we will work methodically through the process of sorting out your wayward clothing collection and getting it back on track.

My ongoing observations also revealed that at around the age of forty, most women have lived through a combination of life experiences, all of which will have influenced their bodies and shape both physically and mentally. Things like meeting a partner, divorce, promotion, career change, career regress, childbirth, relocation, caring for elderly relatives, coping with (own and others) health issues, grief, perimenopause, menopause, and hormone changes, to name a few.

Your clothes are a reminder of these changes, and as wardrobes don't have filters, they will represent both the good and the bad. If you've been hanging onto garments for ten, fifteen or even twenty years, by the age of forty, old garments will buy you a one-way ticket to memory lane and a time when perhaps none of these 'experiences' have happened. If you think about it that way, you'll soon realise that the body and mindset changes you are experiencing now were not there all those years ago – weight issues being a prime example; therefore, if you are still storing old items in your wardrobe that are no longer wearable (due to the inevitable life changes), they are not serving you. In fact, they are more likely to have a negative impact on your mood.

At this point, I want to talk a bit about 'age-appropriate clothing'. When Ted asked me the question, *"Does being forty-plus actually make a real difference?"* I started thinking about women who won't wear certain things because they are 'old'. That led me to wonder what would happen if clothing had no age limits whatsoever—because that is what I believe. How we feel should dictate what we wear, not the number of years since we were born.

Age-appropriate clothing, in my opinion, is a false notion. Sadly, clothing industry marketing strategies categorise clothes into targeted age groups in a bid to increase sales. The fashion industry reigns supreme at this made-up concept of age-appropriate clothing and has done so for years. I, therefore, forgive you if you thought there were such a thing as adult-age labels for clothing, but trust me, there is not.

One thing we cannot ignore when talking about clothing and age, though (particularly in reference to women), is the amount of flesh that is on show.

Silver Curve model and Body Confidence Activist Rachel Peru didn't become a model until the age of forty-six; she wears a UK size 16 (at time of writing this book) and is often seen presenting live in just her underwear. There are those who may frown upon this, but the truth is, there are no rules about how much flesh should be on show. Obviously, when you are out and about, there is an element of common decency and a need to avoid being arrested (!), but besides that, what we wear and how much flesh we show is down to personal choice and **not** our size or our age.

Rachel's story is a compelling one. Her life was a whole lot different in her 20s and 30s when showing her flesh was the very last thing she wanted to do. We're going to learn a bit more about Rachel later on.

As I've said, there are no age-related rules regarding dressing and what we wear. Personally, I can't bear it when I hear terms such as 'dressing youthfully'. There is no such thing. If a person has an enthusiasm for life, they can be described as youthful; it's not clothing that makes that happen.

What *is* true, though, is that you can dress *too old* if you are dated or frumpy. '*Mutton Dressed as Lamb*' is a slang term referring to a dated style or someone who is 'overdressed', someone who is perhaps trying to look younger, better, thinner, happier by courtesy of what they are wearing. It's a false notion – wearing a dated look does nothing except add to a perceived age.

Later in the book we'll go through my cheat sheet which will help you to decide what to do with older (dated) designs and clothing. In the meantime, if you need some kind of mantra to help you make those daily clothing choices, try this one, immortalised by the late Iris Apfel (the woman who lived to be the world's oldest fashion icon).

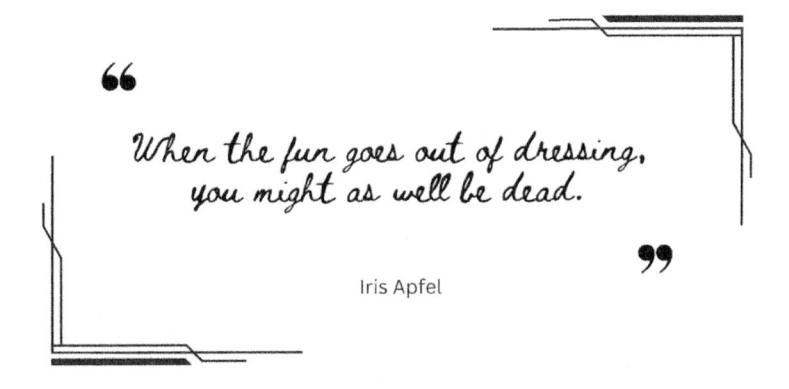

> *When the fun goes out of dressing, you might as well be dead.*
>
> Iris Apfel

If you are unfamiliar with her iconic look, Iris Apfel was known for layering colours and fabrics with tons of oversized jewellery and huge, circular, black-framed spectacles. She became a fashion icon at the grand age of 84 and rocked her look until the day she died aged 102. I think you'll agree that her quote (above) is on point!

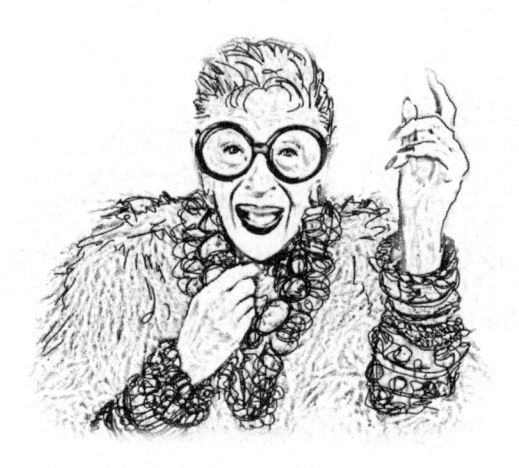

Iris Apfel 29.08.1921 – 01.03.2024

Age & Dressing - Summary

- There is no such thing as age-appropriate dressing rules.
- Individuals are entitled to their own beliefs about what they choose to wear.
- Beliefs around age and dressing stem from an amalgamation of personal thoughts. These include remembering how you used to look, your current mindset, thoughts from others around you, and cultural expectations.
- A dated dress sense can make you look older.

1.4 Body Beautiful Before Clothes

———•———

Earth is the subject of many quotes, poems, and stories because it truly is a breathtaking, beautiful work of art that is too vast, varied, and ever-changing to know fully. There is not an ugly bit of natural earth in existence (except perhaps some parts that have been spoilt by us humans!).

Our bodies are the same. They, too, are the subject of many quotes, poems, and stories because they, too, are truly beautiful. Our bodies are also ever-changing and are unique versions – no two bodies are the same – only comparable in their beauty. So, when we believe that our bodies are as beautiful and breathtaking as the earth, why should we risk sabotaging them by wearing clothes that are subpar?

There are many reasons women feel they cannot clothe their

bodies in the style they want. Sometimes, there are practical considerations, too, which can make the entire process of getting dressed feel like a huge undertaking. In order to dig deeper here, I would like you to take a moment to answer the following questions. They are quick-fire, designed to be answered instantly based on your gut response, and though you may be concerned about the outcome, please don't worry. This is all part of the process of helping you understand how to make the right clothing choices for your body. Ultimately, all of these questions will help to convince you that clothes are not the enemy, in fact, nothing could be further from the truth. Clothes provide our bodies with a second skin of protection and, moreover, arm us with the identity, confidence, look and belief that we choose.

So, deep breath, here goes:

Answer YES or NO.

YES or NO

> Circle ✓ or ✗
> 1. Is your body 10/10? ✓ ✗
> 2. Has your body changed for the better? ✓ ✗
> 3. Do you love your body? ✓ ✗
> 4. Are your clothes 10/10? ✓ ✗
> 5. Have your clothes choices changed for the better? ✓ ✗
> 6. Do you love your clothes? ✓ ✗

If you answered YES to all six questions, then I am delighted for you. Whatever you are doing is working, so keep it up – and continue enjoying your beautiful body and wardrobe.

If – which, let's be honest, is more likely - you answered NO to one or more of these questions (specifically numbers 1-3), then don't panic. Hold tight. The practical guide I will share teaches the principles of owning clothes that bring instant joy and elevate your mood, regardless of body shape or size. Though your feelings towards your body may not change, *it is possible* to change *how you feel* about your clothed self by following this guide.

We all have the power to look great, feel confident and present ourselves in a manner that defines us on our terms – and not on the opinions of others.

The following chapters will also help if you answered NO to any of the questions numbered 4 – 6. My aim is to guide you seamlessly through the process of identifying your best garments, helping you love your clothes and allow them to bring you joy.

> *Disclaimer:* We will not be transforming you into an idea of 'perceived perfection'; the model type with 'perfect hair, body, skin, confidence', etc…because that is not reality. Reality is helping you to use the power of clothes to gain confidence, look good and feel your best, so please, from here on in, try to erase the image of how you believe 'perfection' looks and instead embrace **you** in **your own beautiful entirety**. And don't worry; I am metaphorically holding your hand and cheering you on from the sidelines every step of the way.

> ❝
> *Embracing my body has brought me a sense of contentment and confidence.*
>
> Carole, Company Director
> ❞

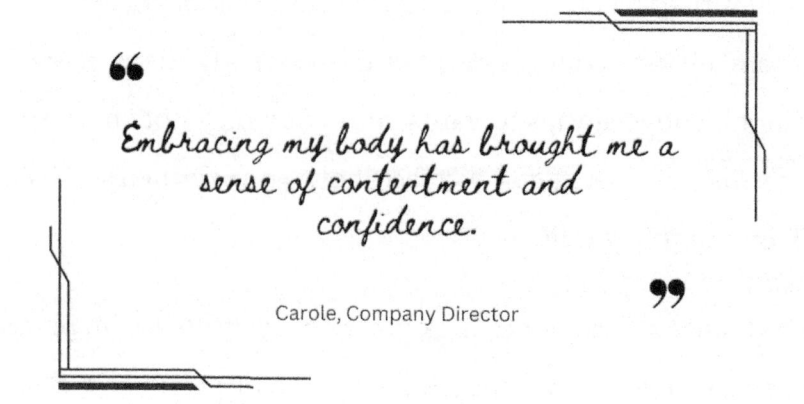

1.5 Switching Focus from Body to Clothes

First impressions. There is countless data around first impressions and how long it takes for us to decide if we like or trust another person purely based on their look. One study suggests that in the first seven seconds, we will form eleven different impressions of a person – simply from their physical appearance. So, let's test it out.

The image below shows five women of various heights and body shapes. Can you guess their clothes sizes?

For now, make a note of your initial thoughts. We will meet them again later, when all will be revealed!

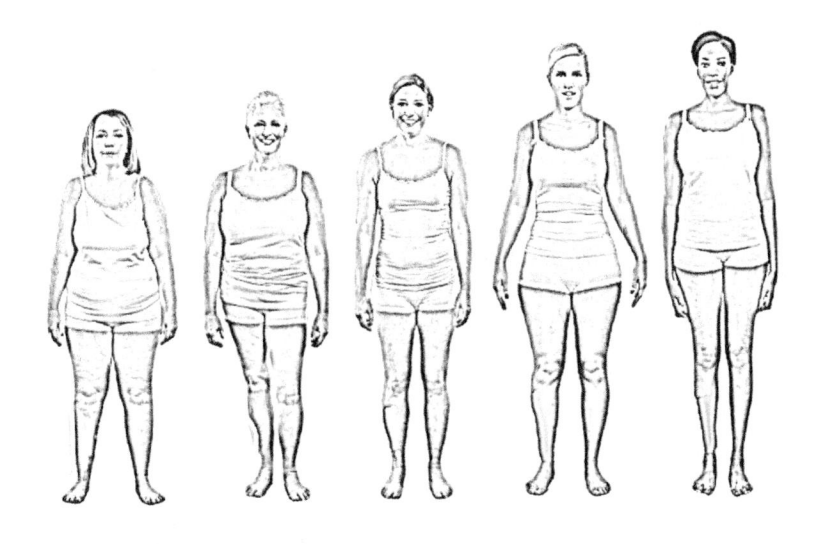

What we're looking at here, really, is the fact that a (well) clothed body has the potential to create a different silhouette and shape compared to our undressed body. The use of (the right) clothing works greatly in our favour, allowing us to exaggerate our best bits and conceal those we'd rather draw attention away from. If we are dressed favourably, not only is our body shape positively affected, but so is our confidence, which means that during those first seven seconds, the eleven impressions will be more upbeat than if we had simply 'thrown something on'.

Silhouette Rather Than Body Shape

It has been the norm for a long time to compare women's body shapes to fruits, such as *apples* and *pears*. Flat angular forms like *triangles* and *rectangles* are also common comparisons, as is the *hourglass*.

There are undeniable flaws in all these terms; however, most obviously, these comparisons refer only to the torso, with no mention of the head, neck, and limbs. These terms remain widely used, though, particularly within the personal styling industry as they are universally understood and can benefit when it comes to matching a general garment shape to a general body shape. If these terms work for you, please don't let me discourage you from using them. I just want to take a moment to dig a little bit deeper.

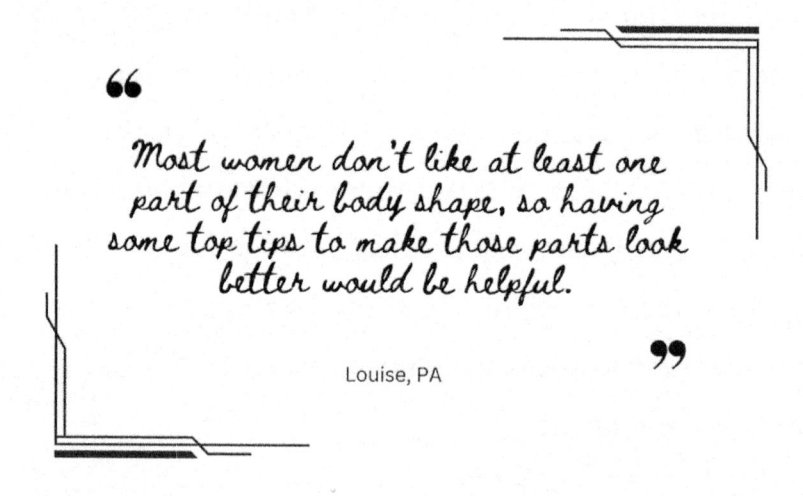

> Most women don't like at least one part of their body shape, so having some top tips to make those parts look better would be helpful.
>
> Louise, PA

'Silhouette' refers to the overall outline shape an outfit creates from head to toe, including footwear. For example, a heel lifts the hem of an outfit further away from the floor, which changes the proportion of the waist to the floor compared to a flat shoe, and thus, the silhouette changes, too.

To become proficient at looking at outfit silhouettes, you will need a full-length mirror and space to step back far enough away to see everything in one go. Only by viewing your entire look will you know how you are seen. If you stand too close to a mirror and cannot see your full length, it creates a tendency to focus on body areas you don't particularly like. When you focus on one area in isolation, then you begin to 'dress' for that 'area', adding clothes or unnecessary layers, which do nothing except attract more attention to that area. Learning to dress your entire body as one (silhouette) will detract focus from the areas you least like.

This is important, so I'm going to say it again:

Learning to dress your entire body as one silhouette will detract focus from the areas about which you are most sensitive.

For example, women who have what I call 'Armitage' – they don't like their upper arms - might cover up by adding an elbow-length bolero cardi over sleeveless items, which simply attracts attention to that very area.

If cover-up items are used but crucially **not considered part of the overall outfit silhouette**, they tell a story, which goes like this:

> "This woman is unhappy with her arms; she doesn't feel comfortable to be seen in her sleeveless garment choice. Presumably she used to like her arms because she owns a sleeveless garment, so why is she unhappy now? Why doesn't she wear something different then? Oh, perhaps she doesn't have anything else to wear, or doesn't like anything in her wardrobe, or maybe nothing fits! Is she too *insert adjective* to think about herself?"

All that from a simple bolero cover-up.

Our clothes are a visual language; they are not two-dimensional objects; they tell a story about who we are, including emotion. It's important to consider what emotion and story our clothes are telling.

To become more silhouette-aware, try this:

1. Look in the full-length mirror and train your eyes to scan your entire dressed shape, checking where your eyes land.
2. If your eyes zoom straight to one area, it suggests your silhouette is not balanced unless you have created an intended focal point to steer your eyes to.
3. Close your eyes. Open them after a few seconds and scan your entire dressed shape again.
4. You will be surprised at what vanishes when you stop focusing on one area and make a habit of looking at your entire form or 'garment silhouette'.

51

5. This is a great habit to develop, so we will have more practice scanning silhouettes when we move on to outfit combinations later in the book.

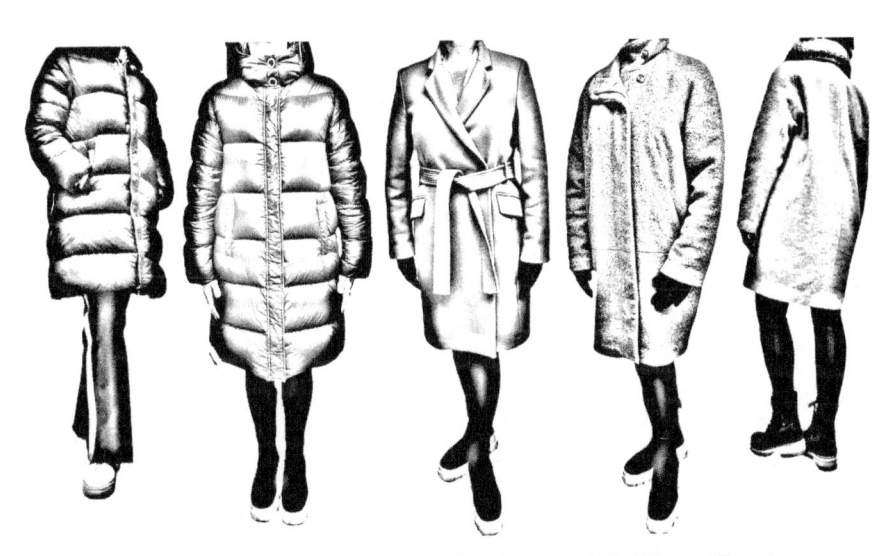

To illustrate, look at these three knee-length coats, which all have different silhouettes. You can see how each reveals or disguises body shape.

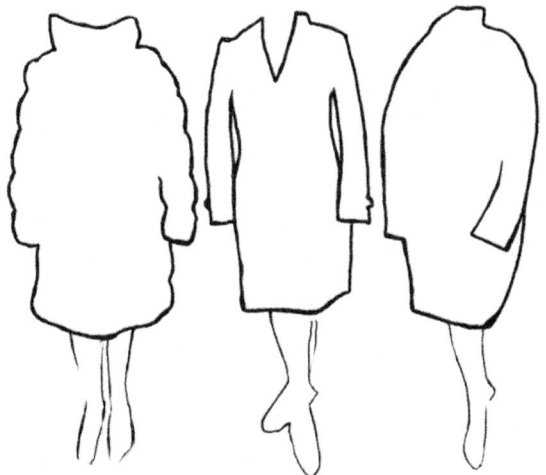

1. Balances shoulder & hips   2. Shows off waist   3. Disguises waist

Garment Proportion Rather Than Body Size

Once you become familiar with the silhouette of your entire body from head to toe, you can start looking at your proportions.

Important: Body proportions are not the same as size. Size is simply a measurement. For example, a 10-inch difference between the bust/hip and waist measurement is depicted as the perfect feminine figure, but if you are short in the body and have long slender legs, your silhouette won't match those measurements, nor will it if you are a woman who is longer in the body and shorter in the leg. Size really is just a number. Proportion is what matters.

The same method you used to identify silhouettes can be used to look at your proportions.

1. Stand in front of a full-length mirror to familiarise yourself with your body proportions.
2. Look at the distance from your shoulders to your waist and then your waist to the floor.
3. Look at your body widths, too. Consider your shoulder width along with your bust, waist and hip width. Remember, you're not measuring; you're simply looking at your proportions.

4. If you are new to the full-length mirror, it can feel a little uncomfortable to stare at yourself, but the mirror is the best tool for helping you recognise clothing shapes that fit and flatter your body.
5. Knowing your body proportions rather than size will make it even easier to find clothes that fit and flatter you.

An easy way to gauge your proportions:

1. Standing in front of a full-length mirror (without shoes), hold your mobile phone out in front of you (portrait). Use your phone as a measure and count how many 'phone heights' tall you are from shoulder to waist and waist to floor.
2. Now, turn the phone sideways (landscape) and count the number of phone widths on your shoulders, bustline, waist, and hips.
3. Next, use the straight edge of your phone to line up your outer hip with your shoulder and see if the angle line (of your phone's straight edge) slopes in towards your body or away from your body.
4. Put on some shoes now and repeat the exercise. Compare the proportion differences between the two.
5. Now you're going to turn sideways and look at your bum, tum and boobs. What sticks out furthest? Use your phone (as above) to measure if you're unsure.
6. Finally, have a look at what you are wearing and compare the proportions of where the garments start

and end. How far from your waist? How far from the floor?

There's no need to log your outcome unless you want to. The point of this exercise is to help you become confident in looking at your body, its proportions, and how just the length or the width of a single garment can change your overall silhouette. I meet women all the time who tell me that they know what their body shape is but don't look at themselves in detail or refuse to look in the mirror at all. This means that they are doing little more than guessing about the fit of their clothes – whether they are too tight, too loose, too long or too short.

It's also important to note that posture directly affects the proportions of our bodies, so it's helpful to check how we're standing. Give this a try:

Check Your Posture

Your proportion will be different if you're not standing up tall and straight.

1. In front of the mirror, stand slightly on your tiptoe so your heel is off the floor, with one foot slightly in front of the other. Resting your front heel on the top of your back foot will stabilise you. This will force you to use

your core to remain central and not lean to one side.
2. With your feet in place, lift your rib cage up and away from your pelvis and roll your shoulders up, back, and down.
3. Retain position, slightly shift your hips forward and hold your chin up high by extending up through the back of the neck.
4. Remember to breathe.
5. Stand in this position and look in your full-length mirror to check your outfit before you leave home.

The more we are aware of our body proportions and how clothes sit on our bodies, the easier it is to tweak length or choose a flattering trouser leg shape. We will also begin to understand where a tops should end and which clothing shapes will create a balanced silhouette for our bodies. *And when we gain all of this knowledge, we begin to control our looks and start to be perceived by others how we wish to be perceived. Remember: seven seconds, eleven impressions.*

56 | 2ND SKIN

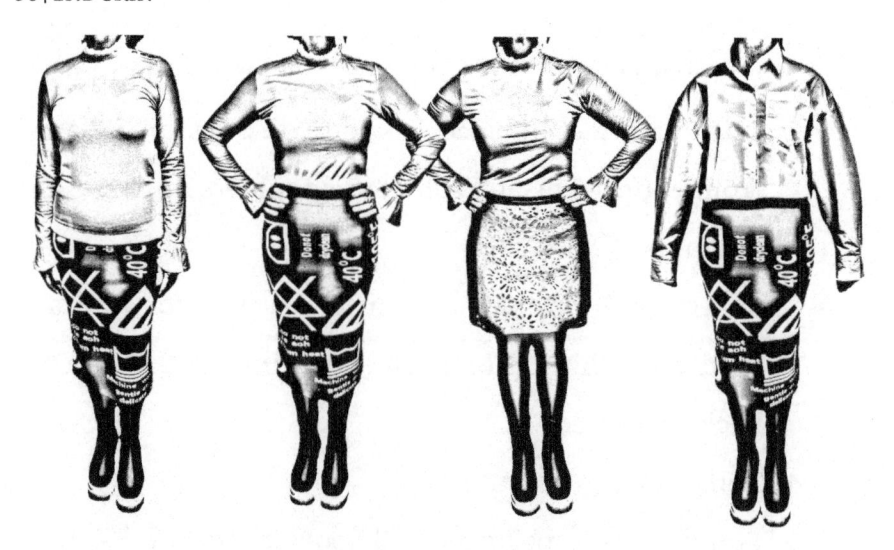

The tops in these 4 outfits have different garment proportions - where the top ends, and width due to fabric fit. Proportion accentuates various body proportions:

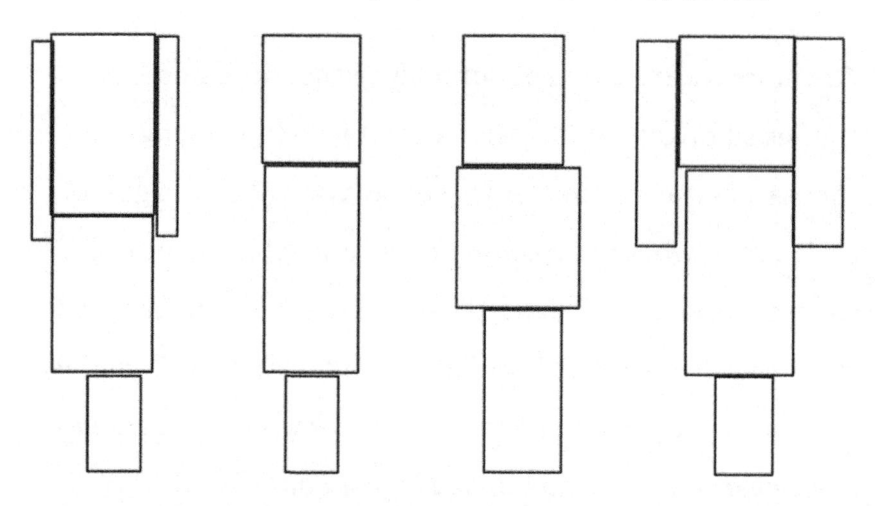

1. Lengthens body   2. Lengthens legs   3. Defines waist   4. Narrows hips

Correct Fit Will Flatter Your Body

The human body is an organic form of proportion, scale, and ratios, with unique curvatures and contours that change with time and lifestyle. What does not change, though, are our *core* proportions. We cannot make our legs longer or our shoulders narrower; our bone frame is fixed. The size and shape fluctuations we experience are caused by increased or decreased muscle mass, fat cell expansion or contraction, droop, medication side effects, and posture-skewing disease. If you think about it, our bodies and their form are so complex that it's a wonder any 'off-the- peg' clothes fit.

In fact, you are correct if you believe that clothes 'simply don't fit'. People often wear ill-fitting clothes or choose stretchy fabrics rather than persevere with the agonising torment of a perfect fit.

In a 2023 Vogue Business Reporter, Maliha Shoaib stated that 46% of e-commerce clothing returns are due to inaccurate sizing. That's almost half! So be reassured. Even the clothing industry can't get it right. No wonder it's a problem for us, the humble consumer, too.

The good news is that now that we've taken the time to really consider our exact body shapes, we are 50% there in terms of our overall clothing solution—which is great.

Keep going! You are well on your way to perfect attire.

Switching Focus From Body To Clothes – Summary

- Understanding your body in terms of silhouette and proportion will help you to match the shape and fit of clothes.
- Clothes that fit properly will flatter your body shape.
- The only way to fully understand your body shape is by regularly looking in a full-length mirror.
- Once familiar with your body's shape, you will find it easier to learn how to recognise balanced silhouettes and use clothing proportions to create outfit shapes that you love.

1.6 Mind Matters

We can talk about past style, age, body shape, and how to look at our bodies in preparation for dressing them; however, mindset can eclipse everything. Every single one of us is on a different journey, and it is fair to say that the results we achieve will be based on what actions (choices) we implement. Mindset is, without question, the biggest influence when it comes to preventing our actions, which means it directly impacts our subsequent results.

If you think or know that 'mind-matter' could be stopping you from taking action and caring about what you wear, here are some suggested solutions:

Mindset towards what you wear covers three areas:

1. Acceptance of your starting point - Your body today (and your current clothes).
2. Matching what you see in the mirror with what others see.

3. Garment Association.

Garment association might sound somewhat woo-woo, but it's simply referencing when an item of clothing reminds you of something else. In exactly the same way that a particular smell or sound can remind you of something different, our clothes, which are our closest possessions – literally – hold memories, too.

When you look in the mirror, you see more than the clothes – you see how they make you feel mixed with how you felt all the other times you wore them. In addition to these feelings, and unlike a smell or sound, clothes are a physical reminder, a measure of instant proof your size has fluctuated, body parts sagged, or skin tone paled perhaps.

Olivia, a recent client, was struggling with her day look. I pulled out a gorgeous navy-blue midi dress from her wardrobe that I knew could fit with her lifestyle. She needed to dress for business meetings in the day and be a relaxed mum attending school events later, so she could simply add a jacket or coat to the dress, perhaps change footwear, and be good to go with just one dress. I genuinely believed that this navy dress was perfect, but Olivia disagreed. She whipped it from my hand and tossed it into the 'charity donation' pile.

I looked at the dress again and pointed out to Olivia that it was in perfect condition and had a good label, meaning she could easily sell it as a prime pre-loved item rather than sending it to charity. In short, she didn't need to give it away.

Moreover, it was a perfect piece to match her body shape and style; however, Olivia was having none of it. It later transpired that the dress had been a gift from a former friend, which reminded her of unpleasantries she'd rather forget. So, no matter how perfect the physical dress was, it had to be out of her life.

This scenario can work in the opposite way, too. Garments that hold great sentiment are often re-worn to retain a long-lost feeling or emotion, even if those items are past their best, a poor fit, or just plain unflattering. It's not unusual to want to hold onto clothes that anchor us to our past or keep us feeling secure. The solution here is to store them away from your daily go-to Wardrobe.

Case Study

Madeleine loved how confident she felt in her workplace attire. As soon as she got dressed for work, her clothes made her feel prepared for whatever her day ahead presented – and it showed. Her posture and body language told everyone she encountered that she was competent and confident at work. Her off-duty and weekend wardrobes, though, were a different story.

Madeleine didn't know how to create that same confidence outside of her workplace wardrobe, even to the point where she would turn down social invites – especially if she knew that a work colleague would be present.

After spending some time with Madeleine, it became clear that her problem was in the way she accessed her wardrobe and bought her clothing. When it came to choosing her off-duty clothes, Madeleine would randomly select garments that she perceived as 'non-work' pieces based on what was presented in fashion articles or what she saw other people wearing. She would also choose 'going out clothing' based on what she believed she was 'expected' to wear from the influence of brand advertising and her perception of the 'accepted norm'.

Unsurprisingly, this 'scattergun' approach resulted in a collection of oddments that were the complete opposite of her stylish work attire—clothes that were simply not her personal style.

I explained to Madeleine that she could retain her confident, chic, clean-line work style clothing shapes and silhouettes out of hours, all she needed to do was adapt elements such as colours, details, fabrics, and accessories. Madeleine's challenge was that she was so focused on her off-duty clothing being completely different to her work attire that she was *moving away from herself and what suited her. Once she understood that she already **had a fab style**, it was simply a matter of 'occasion appropriate' dressing utilising her existing fab style – not completely overhauling her wardrobe. This elevated Madeleine's lifestyle no end.*

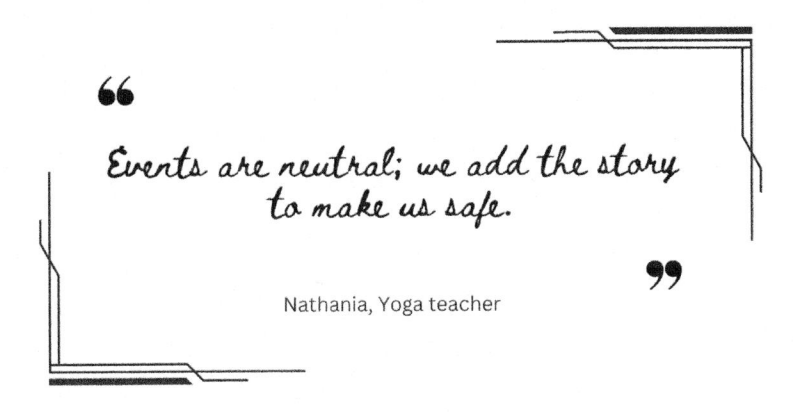

> ❝ Events are neutral; we add the story to make us safe. ❞
>
> Nathania, Yoga teacher

When Things Go Wrong

It is not always possible to tell a woman to accept her starting point, body, and current clothes collection, especially when they contain history and memories.

As I touched upon earlier, self-esteem and body changes, along with mental and physical health, can make it difficult or even impossible at times to be in the right mindset for acceptance.

If this is where you are, take comfort in knowing you are not alone, and help is available. I know, trust, and follow professionals who are experts in the field of supporting and transforming mindsets in order to create space for clarity. Because my expertise begins and ends with wardrobe therapy, I spoke explicitly to five professionals offering different mindset therapies. Here are their words, written in a way which explains exactly how they can offer help and support:

> 1. **Janie is a Holistic Transformation Therapist,** *and I asked if any of her therapies could help women with body confidence. Janie's response was Havening Techniques®. Havening is a method which alters the brain landscape to permanently remove the adverse effects of traumatisation and pathologically stuck emotions. Janie went on to explain that this psycho-sensory therapy is gentle and suitable for most people to do themselves if given the correct guidance. Janie's website offers free advice, online courses, or options to work with her.*

"There will probably be underlying reasons for associations with negative body image or body parts that I would first address, and then I would clear these and replace them with body positivity"
Janie Whittmore

> 2. **Rachel Peru**, *who I mentioned earlier, is a* **Body Confidence Activist and Founder of Liberté Free to Be.** *Rachel changed her own midlife around and now works relentlessly to empower and inspire other women during their mid-years. At age 53 and a UK size 16, Rachel has the confidence to present to a live audience in just her underwear, but believe me when I tell you that this was not the body acceptance she had in her*

20s or 30s. I asked Rachel where this midlife confidence came from, and she told me it was due to a shift in mindset.

One of her stories that resonated with me was when she told me she'd got rid of her weighing scales. Rachel had become incredibly conscious of her weight and began each day by weighing herself. Depending on what the scales read, her mood would be set for the rest of the day – and the next and the next and the next. After a while, Rachel realised that she was letting her weighing scales control her daily mood, meaning that if she didn't get the reading she was hoping for, she would experience a bad day before she'd even had a shower. Getting rid of those scales freed her from their control, and now, through her personal experiences and sheer passion, she helps to amplify the voices of women aged forty and over. She shares her personal stories in a bid to help women live their mid-lives in a way that provides them with the freedom and fulfilment they deserve. If you are at that age, I cannot recommend reaching out to Rachel highly enough. She is 'off the scale' (excuse the pun!) when it comes to helping women to gain and retain a positive mindset.

> **"...now I'm 53 I finally feel at ease with my body which is liberating."**
> Rachel Peru

*3. **Andrea Marsh** successfully changes the mindsets of her clients using treatments that guide them through acceptance of physical body changes. In addition, she helps them to reconnect their bodies with their minds. Her methods include* gut-to-brain access, nutrition, the Hara diagnosis and even laughter diffusion. She is an experienced **Shiatsu Practitioner and Chinese Medicine Therapist.** Andrea's Shiatsu therapy provides a fully clothed touch experience, which involves jiggling the body, buttock pummelling, wobbling the thighs, and feeling around for organ gargling. You can see where the laughter diffusion fits in! Andrea's expertise and knowledge are both incredible and fascinating. Don't take my word for it – Andrea's website offers e-books, videos, and DIY support.

> **"As the treatments went on over the space of 3 months, my client accepted her thighs. Her whole mindset about changing her body had turned around."**
> Andrea Marsh

4. As a Solution-based Psychotherapist and Hypnotherapist, Dipti Tait's mission is to help people navigate the stresses of life calmly, confidently, and successfully.

Dipti goes on to explain that body image acceptance and body dysmorphia exist in the subconscious, and it's the disconnect between body and mind that causes the unfiltered versions of what people believe they see in the mirror. Whether it's Fight – resistance, Flight – run away, or Freeze – rather not deal with it, Dipti's methods will reduce your emotional overwhelm to overcome fear using the powerful intelligence of hypnotic trance. Her deeply soothing hypnotic relaxation method of Free Flow Transformation Therapy® will help you find calm contentment so that you can turn problems into solutions.

"The mind and body are connected, and the more you understand

*how the mind works, the better relationship
you will have with your body."*
Dipti Tait

5. Jessica is an Integrative Health Practitioner and Health Coach *who uses functional medicine lab testing to help you get to the root cause of imbalances in your body. She explains how weight gain is often a symptom of chronic stress, hormone imbalances and pathogens. As an expert in perimenopause and menopause, she uses your data and symptoms to craft a holistic plan to get your mind and body back into balance.*

"When you are grateful for your amazing body, you're much more likely to pay attention to what she's telling you through symptoms. It's then that it becomes easy to make the changes in your life that help you feel vibrant"
Jessica Green

You Are Your Own Worst Critic

As I began to build a bank of images to accompany this book, I approached women and asked them for permission to take anonymous photos of them wearing clothes from their existing wardrobes. The purpose was to showcase outfit silhouettes and proportions on a broad selection of bodies rather than using images of professional models. This was to provide authentic representations that would resonate with readers.

Every picture is headless, and the only information given in each image is the woman's height and typical UK dress size. After taking the photos, I selected the ones I wished to use, removed the backgrounds or made them neutral, and then sent them back to each woman for their approval prior to final use.

That was when something amazing happened.

Each image was instantly approved, but more than that, they were all accompanied by the added message:

"I look better than I thought."

It is generally accepted that people recognise each other by their faces. When we look in the mirror, we will recognise ourselves and compare and contrast our faces for signs of changes to our appearance, tiredness, dark eyes, or anxiousness… any one of several expressions and moods. It is this that will be at the forefront of our minds when we are looking in the mirror and working out what to wear.

What I discovered was that by isolating the women's outfits and returning the photos to them without their faces, every single one suspended their usual facial judgment. Instead, they focused on their bodies and what they were wearing, which made them a lot more comfortable. They even embraced their clothing and loved their style.

Women think they can't wear something because it doesn't look good enough, yet the truth is that what *we* see in the mirror is not the true reflection of what *other people* see. When we look in the mirror, whilst we think we are looking at our physical and outward appearance, and indeed we are, what we are *also* seeing is this physical reflection mixed (and perhaps contaminated) with our thoughts, feelings, moods and inner voice. Thus, when the same reflection was returned to the women in the photographs a few days later – minus their faces – their reaction was much more positive. Their response was no longer tainted by other emotions.

My sister taught me an exercise she learned from a psychologist, which was designed to help whenever she found herself in a situation with multiple answers and was unclear about which one to pursue. The psychologist told her to do the following:

1. Draw an outline of a person.
2. Write down what she **thought** she should do in the head section.
3. Write down what she **wished** she could do in the torso section.

4. Tear the paper to remove the head, leaving only the torso.
5. That, then, is the answer.

I didn't realise just how true this was until I took these headless photos. As we delve deeper into the book, you'll see some of these photographs, so I want to take a moment to point out that every model—for that is what they are—is wearing her own clothes from her own wardrobe at the time of the photo.

Here's something you can consider, following on from what I've just revealed:

If you own clothes that you are not wearing, is it because there are other thoughts in your head stopping you from doing so?

As Henry Ford once said,

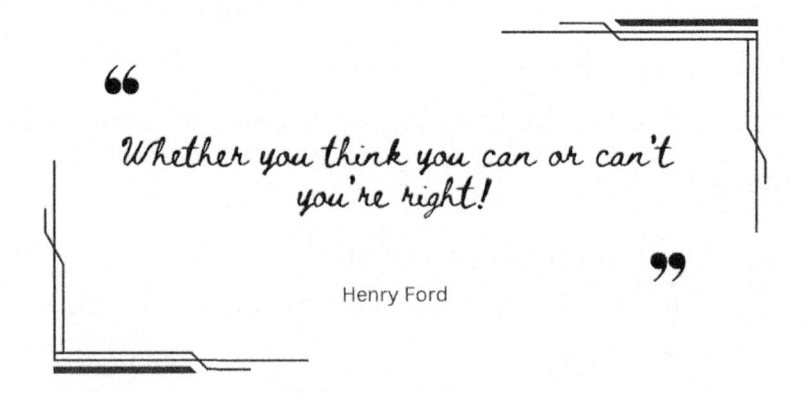

> Whether you think you can or can't you're right!
>
> Henry Ford

So, think you *can* and wear your best outfit today.

Talking about body perception, remember the ladies from the Body Beautiful illustration earlier? It's time to reveal the answer to their sizes and one other interesting fact:

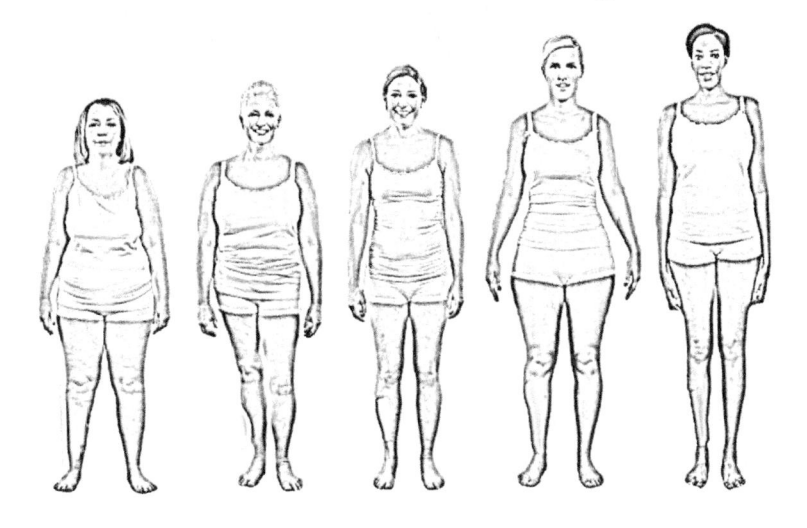

5'2" Size14 | 5'4" Size18 | 5'8" Size12 | 5'11 Size12 | 6'1" Size10

Different shapes and sizes, BUT all exactly the same weight!

Hopefully you can see that weight bears little resemblance to what size a woman wears. It is all about body shape and proportion.

Let's take that further and look at some outfits that are considerate of proportion and silhouette rather than size. Notice here how the shorter length of the top and the wider hem of the jeans, along with heeled footwear, add the illusion of height. For reference, I have added the women's heights and dress sizes below each image.

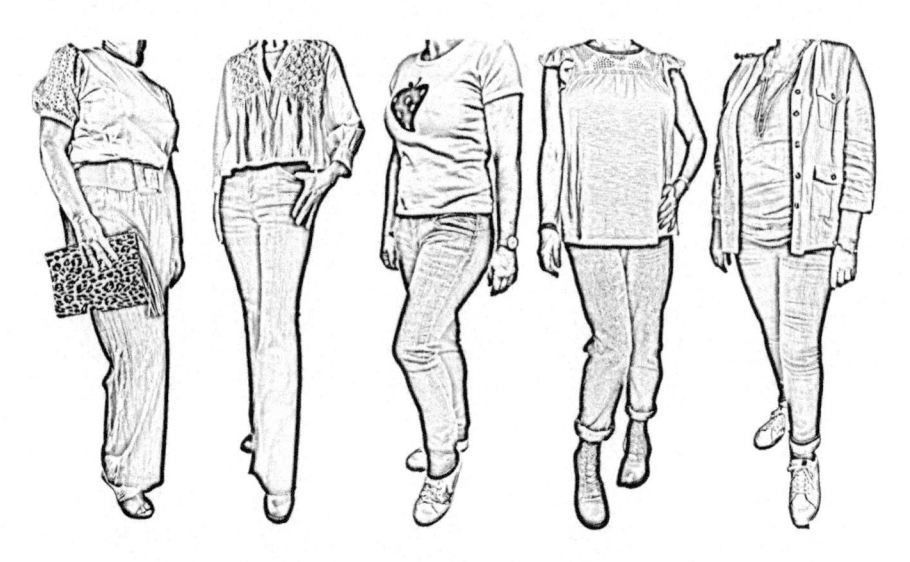

5'5" Size 14 | 5'0" Size 8 | 5'5" Size 12 | 5'3" Size 12 | 5'11" Size 20

Mind Matters – Summary

- Body acceptance is not about trying to prevent change from happening or disguising the signs of age. It's about embracing new beginnings, enjoying what you've already learnt, and looking forward to what is next. Then you will shine with style.
- Fashion doesn't reflect your body shape because it is marketing and selling, not styling. Once your mindset turns to your needs rather than marketing, it becomes easier to accept. (I doubt we are going to get a shop marketing a slogan for over-40s with a middle-aged spread anytime soon, and nor would we want that!).
- Holding onto clothes you've had for years because you

believe you love them or they will fit again one day, often has a negative effect. This is because they can become a reminder of the age and time when you bought and wore them, and perhaps highlight changes that you are unlikely to ever reverse. Move the negative size or life reminders out of your go-to wardrobe and focus on what makes you feel good today.

- If how you feel about your body laid bare is preventing you from having wardrobe joy and wearing clothes that give you confidence, please look up the experts mentioned. I have listed them again below. Each has an online offering and will be able to guide you or help you to find the support you need.

Janie - Holistic Therapies – janiewhittemore.com
Rachel - Body Confidence Activist - liberteltd.com
Andrea - Shiatsu & Chinese medicine - cotswoldmenopause.co.uk
Dipti – Psychotherapy & Hypnotherapy - diptitait.com
Jessica - Menopause Expert - jessicagreenwellness.com

Phew! What a journey. I hope you are enjoying all you have learned so far and are beginning the (tentative) process of acceptance of yourself and your beautiful body.

We're now moving on to talk about clothes in more detail, so remember, once clothed, we usually like our bodies more than we initially thought we would – just like my headless models did!

See you in the mirror!

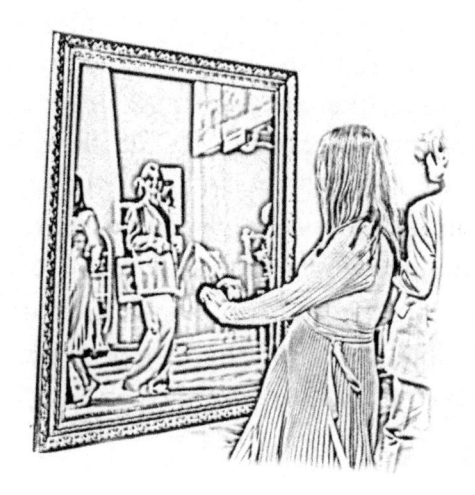

2. Clothes Unpicked

---•---

Our bodies are clothed almost immediately after birth, and, as we've discovered in Chapter 1, they evolve with age. This is not dissimilar to what happens on Earth's surface. Covered by nature and infrastructure, it evolves in accordance with what is required of it, adapting as it ages. External factors such as the climate affect how it looks, as do the environment and materials available for its development. Earth also has the capacity to rebuild itself after natural disasters, so just as this beautiful natural World aligns its surface to life, we can align our clothing to the needs and demands of our lifestyle journey.

When it comes to clothes, the more you understand them from different aspects such as fabric, cut, versatility, characteristics, and cost, the more informed your clothing choices will be in preparation for your body and lifestyle changes. In this chapter, you will learn that clothes are so much more than what we see on the hanger. It's a lesson in clothing if you like, but without a test, though the reward is great. By the end of this chapter, you will have discovered new ways to detach yourself from clothes that are not right for you and narrow down the search for clothes that are perfect. If you want to save shopping time, reduce fashion faux pas, and ooze more style, then it's time to learn about clothes.

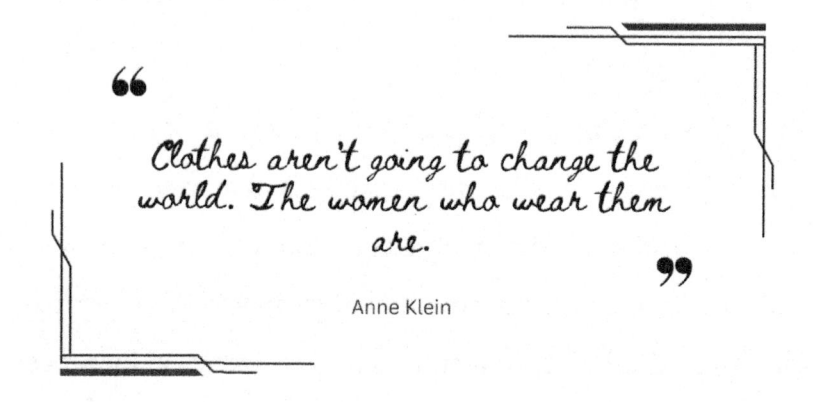

> **"**
> *Clothes aren't going to change the world. The women who wear them are.*
> **"**
>
> Anne Klein

2.1 - Fabric & Cut

Identical garments in different fabrics do not look the same, and it isn't just colour and pattern variants that cause it. The main difference comes from the properties of each individual fabric.

Here's a simple way to understand this concept:

- Starting with colour, visualise a pair of soft khaki green cargo pants. Think work-from-home or safari holiday vibes.
- Now picture the same cargo pants in neon yellow and switch your holiday vibe focus to Ibiza.
- Next, add a variant of fabric property, perhaps a thin yet crisp-to-the-touch parachute-like fabric. Instantly, you will see the famous cargo pants Mel B wore on the Spice Girls movie tour in the '90s.

Every one of these scenarios is based on a pair of cargo pants, but the outcome of their overall look and feel could not be more different.

Learning the full complexity of fabric properties and fibre

composition is not necessary at this stage; however, if you do have a specific interest in this area, please see the details for my Clothing Fit & Fabric Course at the end of the book. This course provides much more information on fabric and fibre composition.

What *is* worth knowing at this point is how different fabrics hang or sit on your body, how fabrics feel, and what silhouette a garment makes in different fabrics. When you understand this, you can competently describe clothes in the fit and shape you like.

Let's start by taking a second to describe the fabrics of each garment you are currently wearing. Say it out loud, in your head, or jot it down. Whatever works for you.

Now, look at the following points – did you answer any of these questions in your description?

1. How does the fabric feel to touch? soft, crisp, thick, stiff, floppy etc.
2. Does the fabric cause your body to react? sweat, itch, cool, cosy etc.
3. What silhouette does the hang of the fabric create? floaty, rigid, clingy etc.

Whilst you may not have given it much thought, your

experience of handling and wearing clothes from the day you were born will already have created discoveries and personal preferences around fabrics and style. Some you will have decided you don't like because they irritate your skin, for example.

To delve into the details of how to identify your best clothing fabrics, four main characteristics affect the wearability and shape of the garment, along with its hang and fit to your body:

1. The stiffness of a fabric.
2. The drape of a fabric.
3. Fabrics that are stretchy or have elasticity.
4. Non-stretch fabrics that are rigid or described as woven fabrics.

An example of **stiff fabrics** can be seen in garments like a classic denim jacket or the collar and cuffs of a tailored shirt. To identify a garment made from stiff fabric, take a corner of the waistband or shoulder and then hold it out at arm's length away from you, between your thumb and index finger. A garment made from stiff fabric will retain some shape rather than just go floppy.

A garment made from **fabric with a drape** does the opposite. Picture a fine silk scarf that can be pulled from a small space, such as a magician's fist, yet resembles the vast size of a parachute. That is a highly drapey fabric. Holding a garment with high draping fabric between your thumb and forefinger will hang like an elegant fluid slither. If you imagine a drapey fabric made into a classic denim jacket, for example, it would resemble a blouse. Equally, think about the reams of silky, drapey fabric used to make a full-length voluminous ball gown, then switch the exact same amount of fabric for denim. (Remember the magician's fist full of silk? Denim wouldn't fit in his hand). The ball gown skirt made from the same amount of stiff denim fabric would protrude like a giant tutu and not resemble an elegant ball gown precariously sweeping the ground.

So, in essence, stiff fabrics hold their shape and are typically used for tailoring classic jeans and blazers. Examples of stiff fabrics are leather, cotton canvas, and crunchy cotton shirts. Drapey fabrics, on the other hand, are typically used for garments like floaty dresses, long-flowing skirts, soft chiffon blouses, and super wide pants (trousers).

Many fabrics fall within the spectrum between the stiffness of classic denim and the drape of fine silk. If you popped into your wardrobe right now and tested each garment with your thumb and forefinger, you would find yourself commenting that most are *"not as stiff as denim, and not as drapey as silk"*.

Don't worry about this, though. The fact that they don't fit into either stiff or drapey isn't an issue, and it will all make more sense when we move onto aligning clothes with lifestyle and body shape.

Need a visual example of the real garments? Scan the QR code to be taken to the digital outfit library and click on the image titled Chapter 2.1

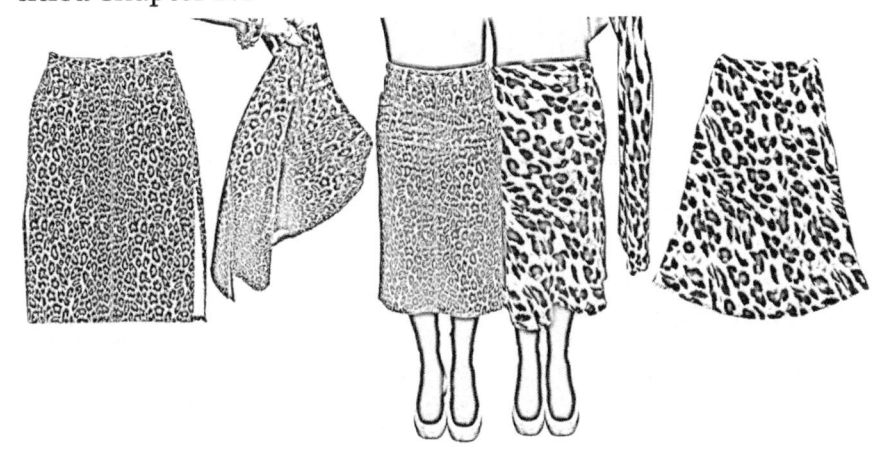

Stiff Fabric and Drape Fabric

SCAN TO VIEW REAL WOMEN OUTFIT LIBRARY

After stiff and drapey, the next two fabric characteristics are **rigid (or non-stretchy)** and **stretchy**. Though these are characteristics in their own right, both can also be found in stiff and drapey fabrics. If you had difficulty identifying stiff or drapey clothes in your wardrobe, it could be because they are stretchy, too.

An example of a garment made from high-stretch fabric is gym leggings. Most gym leggings are now made in a 4-way stretch fabric to enable expansion and retraction of the most excessive body movements (such as motion-flow yoga) without bursting a seam. A pair of trousers as tight fitting as leggings in a non-stretch-rigid fabric would make it impossible for the body to do the same range of movement *without* bursting a seam!

You may even have experienced a situation where you've lowered your hips into a seated position and felt the tightening of fabric over your derriere, causing your back waistband to pull down a little deeper. Then you've heard the distinct sound of a rip and have prayed that nothing too embarrassing is exposed until you can identify where the tear is.

Garments made from rigid fabrics that fit close to the body are cut differently than stretchy garments. Extra-fit seams and the addition of darts are required to create a 3D body shape, and a fastening is needed to get the garment on and off. Stretchy garments, by contrast, can usually be pulled on and off the body without opening or undoing any fastenings.

A stretch element also allows clothing to fit around variants in body size because the fabric can expand. When it comes to the 'cut' of an item of clothing, it is important to understand the difference between stretch and rigid fabrics. It is much harder to achieve the perfect fit in clothing made from rigid fabrics.

This doesn't mean if you struggle with clothes fitting properly, your only option is to settle for stretchy pull-on clothes. Nowadays, there are just as many clothes made from fabrics which are predominately rigid but have an element of stretch for comfort and fit purposes. These fabrics will look just like rigid fabric and lend themselves to the same types of garments, such as jeans, tailoring, and formal dresses, but the element of stretch enables a more snug and comfortable fit without the worry of bursting a seam. Win-win!

Let's think about skinny jeans as an example. Clothing manufacturers add elastic yarn to produce look-a-like denim, which makes jeans stretchy for a skin-tight fit.

Other outcomes are jeans made from thick, stretchy fabrics dyed indigo-denim. They are then decorated with rows of orange top stitching to mimic what is typically associated with the look of classic denim.

Adding elastic to rigid fabrics is seen in most off-the-peg high-street garments, making clothes easier to fit into, especially in the trouser department. Generally speaking, garments made from fabric with high stretch are more casual-looking and cheaper to produce. The more rigid the garment fabric, the more sewing techniques are required to produce it, making it a more expensive item of clothing.

The shape of a stretchy and rigid-stretch garment can look identical, although the ease of wear and overall style will differ.

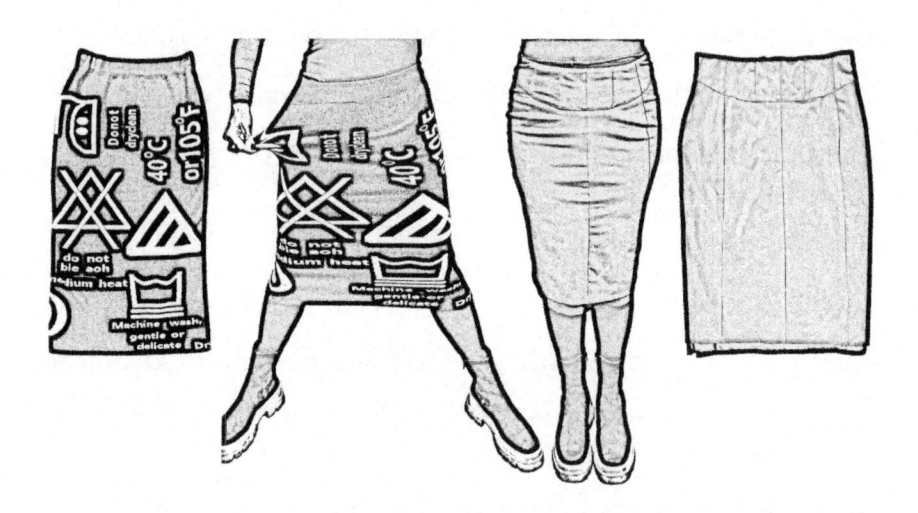

Stretch Fabric and Rigid Fabric

The Stretch Tube Skirt widens as the legs move, whereas the Rigid Pencil skirt narrows just when in situ on a 3D person. It is lined and has a zip fastening.

Some rigid fabrics appear to be a little bit stretchy but don't actually contain elastic. In this instance, the fabric is changing shape on the diagonal (due to its cut) and doesn't spring back to shape like true stretch fabric. This movement is known as 'give'. An example of how this diagonal 'give' affects clothes can be seen when you sit down for a period of time in a snug-fitting skirt and then stand up a while later to notice the fabric around the bum area has gone baggy. The rigid skirt fabric in this example has been pulled taut (including in a diagonal direction) whilst seated as it curves around the body. Because it doesn't contain elastic, there are no 'spring back' properties. Additionally, the body's warmth against the seat acts like an iron and presses it into the seat shape. Whilst this doesn't sound ideal, the 'give' in this fabric allows space for the body to breathe and comfortably move throughout the day without the concern of ripping seams.

Cut On The Bias

Some garments are deliberately designed to take advantage of diagonal fabric 'give' and are referred to as being 'cut on the bias'. Typical bias-cut garments are satin slip dresses, knee-length skirts and camisole tops. In the earlier image of the two leopard print skirts comparing stiff and drape fabrics, the drapey skirt is cut on the bias. Bias-cut garments are great for achieving a close fit over hips, bum, and boobs, without the need for shaping darts and fastenings. This means that if a stretchy fabric feels too clingy or casual, yet a rigid fabric is too tailored or formal, bias-cutting could be the solution.

There is a catch, though. Only a few garment styles can be successfully cut on the bias. The nature of fabric movement means it does not lend itself to design details, structured shapes or garment features like pockets, cuffs, or collars. Seams are kept to a minimum, so if the garment is not made to the highest standards, seams can be unsightly and lumpy, even to the untrained eye.

Now that we've covered the four main fabric types, let's have a look at what else you will find in your wardrobe.

Knits & Jerseys

Jumpers and sweaters. These knits have their own fabric category, made by looping yarn together, just like you would see on knitting needles. The result is a soft, bouncy finish.

Cashmere and wool are very much associated with knits -

cashmere is a luxury fabric that is lightweight yet still super warm.

Jersey is comprised of a very fine knit made by machine and is the fabric most often used for 'T-shirts'. Both knit and jersey have an element of expansion due to the looping method of production which does make them prone to misshape. If you've ever worn a t-shirt top that fits snugly in the morning and becomes baggy over the course of the day, you will have experienced this misshaping. Popping it through the wash will usually bring it back to shape. If you want to avoid this, try looking for garments with either elastane or Lycra® on the label. These spring back into shape and do not get baggy whilst wearing.

Sweatshirts, hoodies and loungewear are made from jersey fabric, too. Typically designed as oversized or slouchy, the shape of these garments means that they don't need to be cut to fit the body.

From what I've shared, you can see that different fabrics behave in different ways, meaning they lend themselves to particular clothing and garments. The variation of fabric types is endless, along with differentiations in the cut, and then you can add pattern, texture and thickness elements to the mix, all of which understandably leads to confusion for most of us. What we are presented with is a mass of clothing styles, shapes, sizes, cuts, weights, colours, patterns ... so by knowing which fabrics you prefer and identifying cuts that flatter your body shape, you can narrow your search for ideal garments considerably.

Choosing Your Clothing Fabrics

You could be forgiven for thinking it would be much easier to choose stretchy fabrics, especially if you have gained a bit of weight and don't want to go up a dress size, but be wary - stretchy is not always flattering. Stretchy garments rely solely on your body shape to provide the garment shape, so there are no disguising parts you may be more sensitive to. Stretchy tops cling, expose bra strap indentation lines and highlight belly rolls, whilst stretchy bottoms expose visible panty lines (VPL) and tend to hang shapelessly.

Rigid fabrics, though, can offer a bit of support. They can hold in a bit here and push up a little there. The fabric can create a more defined silhouette, such as shoulder angles, defined necklines, and a hemline shape, all of which give the illusion of a slicker body frame if fitted well. *Caution*: If your personal style is loose and oversized, the stiffer the fabric, the further away from the body it will hang, which adds width or bulk.

When stretch and rigidity are mixed, you have more power to control fit. A little stretch also prevents fabric wrinkling or creases.

Get the drape and proportions right whilst loving the fabric you've chosen, and every piece in your wardrobe has the potential to be 10/10.

We will look at how to use what we've just covered in Chapter 5.

Choosing Your Clothing Cut

Do not rule out a garment style that you love because it didn't look how you expected it to on the first try. Go back to the two key elements of clothing fit: how the fabric lies on your body and frame and how the garment is cut to move with your body and frame. It could be just a tweak of one of these elements, so try a different fabric or a similar cut before ruling it out completely.

Fit is all about how the garment is cut. The simpler the cut (side seams only and no darts), the more the shape relies on your body to shape it. Remember, too stretchy equals clinginess and exposure to every lump and bump; too stiff and oversized equals unnecessary volume.

The more advanced the cut, the more you can disguise and hide your body. I find it interesting listening to clients talk about cut because it's not always what they mean. They often refer to how the fabric is hanging off or clinging to their body, which is fabric type as opposed to cut. Think back to fine silk and stiff denim. The same cut garment in a different fabric will hang differently—it's not always the cut; it could be the fabric type.

Again, we will delve a little deeper into this area when we reach Chapter 5.

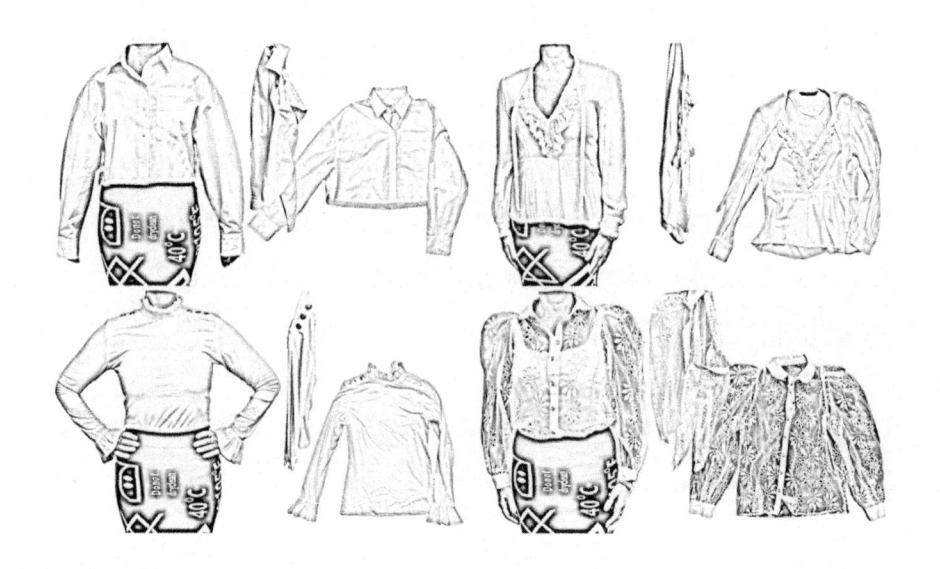

White shirts - different fabrics & different cuts

Top Left - **Stiff Fabric** - Holds garment shape well, is good for collars and cuffs, and hides the middle of the body.

Top Right – **Drapey Fabric** – Floppy garment shape, which is good for fashion details such as frills, flounce and neckties. It skims the body to show curves and body shape without clinging.

Bottom Left – **Stretchy Fabric** – Hugs the body, expanding over curves for an ultra-snug yet comfortable fit. Not suitable for fashion details, just a trim around the neckline and cuff.

Bottom Right – **Rigid Fabric** – Good for lots of garment detailing. The shoulders are highly gathered to create lift and shape, the fabric has been embroidered and laser cut all over, and it is versatile enough to add contrast fabrics to the same garment such as stiffer fabrics for collar and cuff detail.

Clothing Cut And Fit – Summary

- Familiarising yourself with fabric and cut can affect how your clothes fit.
- Well-fitting clothes can make all the difference when it comes to how stylish or polished your finished look is – and this applies to effortless, relaxed looks as well as smarter occasion wear.
- *Clothes that fit properly are more comfortable than ill-fitting clothes in a bigger size.*
- The more you touch, look, describe, and assess the hang of a fabric, the better you will know what types of clothes suit your style and flatter your body shape.

Suggested Actions

Practise feeling and describing fabrics.

1. Start with your favourite garments.
2. Describe the fabric and how each garment works with your body.
   What does it look and feel like? Textured, smooth, soft, sheet etc.
   What is the fabric characteristic? Stretchy, rigid, drapey, stiff etc.
   How does it behave on the body? Clingy, baggy, fitted, etc.
3. Look at how each garment is made to familiarise yourself with the cut:
   What is the fastening type, or is it pull-over/slip-on?
   Does it have darts or panels as well as side seams?
   Any design features like pockets, collars, gathers, trims, sleeves, etc?

Note Writing Space

2.2 Garments vs Outfits

Up to this point, we have referred to both *garments* and *outfits*, but what is the difference, or are they one and the same?

Think of it like this: A flowerbed is just a patch without flowers. A swimming pool is just a pit without water. A garment is just an item of clothing – until it is styled and combined with other garments, footwear and accessories. Then, it becomes a complete outfit.

One garment alone is not a wearable outfit. Even a 'one-and-done' item, such as a dress or jumpsuit, requires footwear at the very least. All your pieces need to be part of a styled outfit combination, so yes, there *is* a difference between a *garment* and an *outfit*.

Do you have garments that you love but don't wear because:

1. You have nothing to wear them with?
2. You only have one thing to wear it with?
3. You can only wear it on days you feel confident?
4. You think it is only suitable for a specific occasion?
5. You have worn it to work, so can't you wear it out of work?
6. You bought it for a wedding so can't wear it anywhere else?

Your daily wardrobe should contain items that can be worn in a choice of styled outfit combinations.

For example, your perfect-shape dress can be paired with a slouch knit, opaque tights, and boots for an Autumnal look. Then, switch the boots for trainers and the knit jacket for a distressed denim jacket to create a Spring look. Style it with bare legs, sandals, and long-beaded necklaces for a Summer feel, or even add flip-flops and a bikini for holiday wear.

Then, there are accessories to consider. A bag or scarf can offer more looks. A floaty chiffon scarf that blows in the breeze or a chunky Winter warmer depending on weather, season, or occasion.

Here are 5 Styling options for one dress from Summer to Autumn:

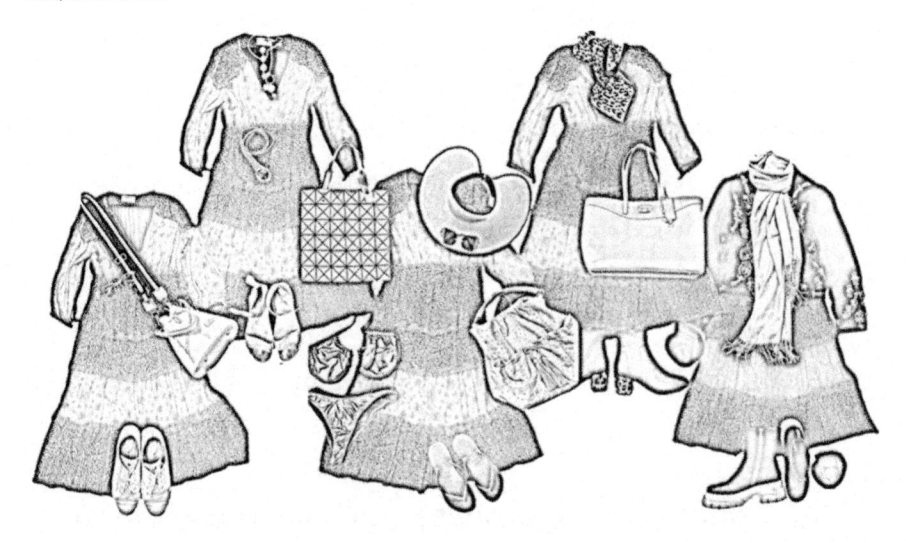

Boho Dress Styled Across Seasons & Occasions

Daily dressing requires your wardrobe to be a bank of ready-to-wear outfits. Choosing an outfit is an easier, quicker and happier way to start your day than picking out a single garment and trying to decide what to pair it with. Figuring out outfit combinations on the spot, particularly if the weather or your plans change, is time-consuming and stressful, and most of all, stagnant if you only have one way of wearing a particular piece.

In the same way we looked at five different ways to wear the same dress, here's an example of seven outfits created from just one pair of trousers. By switching tops, footwear, outer layers, and accessories, you can see how one garment has the potential to make many outfits. We'll be doing this with your garments in Chapter 6.

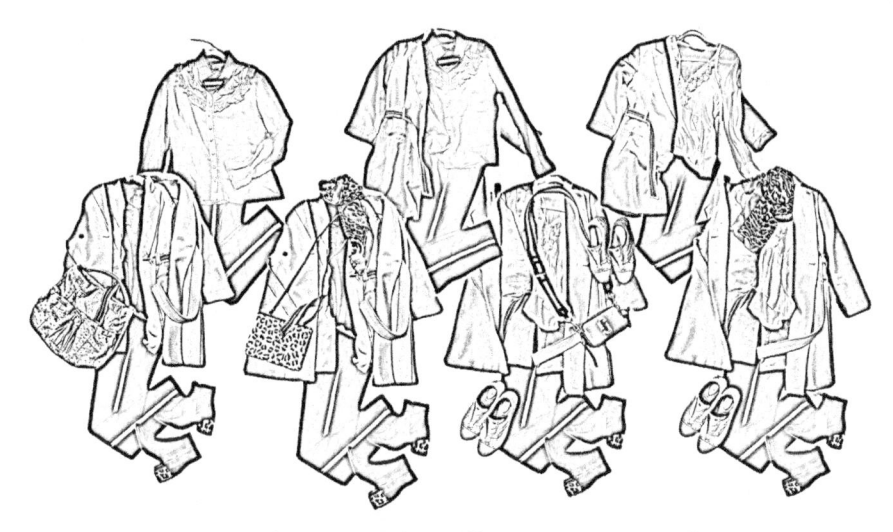

One pair of trousers styled in 7 different ready-to-wear outfits.

Building multiple outfit combinations requires your wardrobe to contain a mix of tops, bottoms, dresses or jumpsuits, outer layers, footwear, and accessories. Not every piece needs to be a statement—outfits are a balance. This means your wardrobe will need to contain some 'Wardrobe Basics'.

'Wardrobe basics' include items such as: layering vests, long-sleeve t-shirts, overlayers for when it's cold, go-to plain dresses or jumpsuits, everyday jeans and an assortment of tights and leggings. Nothing in your 'wardrobe basics' should be out of the ordinary or particularly related to personal style; however, be careful not to fill your wardrobe with too many of these.

It is so easy to let basic garments take over your clothing collection but remember that outfits are a balance, and too many basics will erase your outfit style.

To avoid this, do not select garments solely based on *function*. Think about the colours and fit as well as their functionality. Perhaps consider detailed neck and cuff finishes too. There is such a rich variety of functional garments out there now that you can still consider your taste when choosing your wardrobe basics.

Garments Vs Outfits – Summary

- A single garment is not beneficial to your clothes collection unless it is part of an outfit.
- For a collection of clothes to serve you well, your wardrobe should contain a choice of ready-to-wear outfits that can be worn in several looks and adapted for season, weather and occasion.
- To create multiple outfit combinations, your wardrobe needs to contain a mix of tops and bottoms, one-pieces, layers, outer layers, and footwear.
- Not every piece needs to be overly stylised; however, an imbalance of functional wardrobe basics without consideration for your taste will make it hard to identify your personal style.
- Think style basics, not wardrobe basics, and then each item you own will become more versatile.
- Adapt your ready-to-wear outfits by switching

out footwear, adding outer layers and considering alternative accessories like handbags, scarves, and jewellery.
- **By training your brain to think in outfits, not garments, you will be training yourself to choose well.**

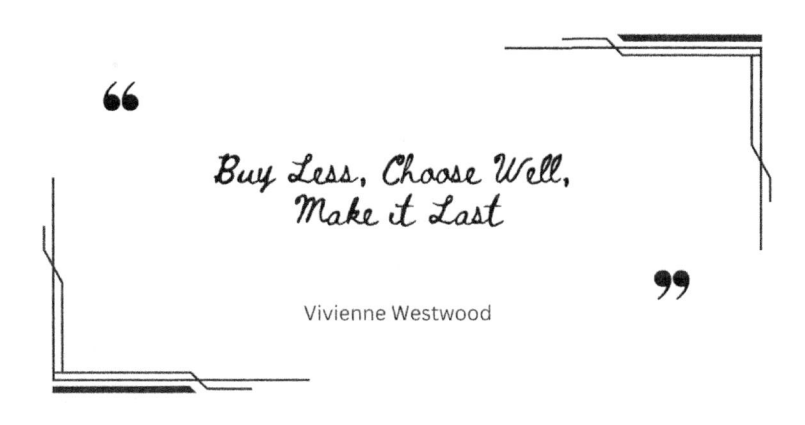

> *Buy Less, Choose Well, Make it Last*
>
> Vivienne Westwood

Suggested Actions

Find your Style Basics

Use the following list to tick off what you already own, and circle those you don't own but think you would like. Be true to yourself - if a garment type isn't your thing, don't tick or circle it. The fewer ticks and circles, the easier it will be to focus on your Unique Personal Style (UPS).

1. Style Basic Jackets

A Jacket shows that you have put thought into your style and communicates that you care about what you do. It works as a stylish layer both day and night and fits under an outer coat:

Unstructured Jacket – soft tailoring or a swing jacket, zipped or buttoned.

Blazer – can have a contrast lining and/or cuffs turned back to reveal lining.

Wrap Jacket – with or without a belt, belts can be switched out or tied back.

2. Style Basic Cardigans or Cardi-gone

A cardigan must do more than resemble a school uniform, so it needs to have a stylish feature. Functionality and colour alone do not make a stylish look and should definitely be referred to as *cardi-gone*:

Cardi Coat – shaped and sized like an outer coat in a knit or jersey fabric.

Short Cardi – sits just on or above the waist and has a full-length sleeve.

Chunky Knit Cardi – Replaces a coat or jacket and looks sumptuous and rich.

3. Style Basic Sweaters

Sweaters do not hide your shape; they exaggerate it and should not be your garment of choice if worn as a cover-up:

Fine Knit or Cashmere – worn with an underlayer that shows the collar/neckline and cuffs to edge the sweater.

Fine Knit or Cashmere Roll-neck – for layering or paired with statement pieces.

Crochet or Open Weave – to show skin or contrast colour underneath.

Chunky Knit – Oversized, sumptuous, and paired with winter *accessories.*

4. Style Basic Trousers

Aka the pant. Your body shape and personal style will determine your chosen style/s here. Matching your ankle diameter with your thigh diameter makes your thighs look thinner. To check if your trousers meet this test, simply lay them out flat and then fold the ankle hem up to the thigh and see if they are equal in width:

Boot Cut or Flare – skims the thigh, in at the knee, wider at the ankle.

Wide Leg – glamorous and dramatic, good for tall women and women with hips & small waists if you style to show your waist.

Skinny Leg – not so good on big thighs unless the outfit is balanced with footwear and an appropriate top or choose a cigarette pant (narrow legs that are slightly narrower at the bottom and finish at or just above the ankle) instead.

Straight Leg – better suited to slim legs; refer to note above about ankle hem and thigh diameters.

5. Style Basic Skirts

To avoid a dated rectangle shape, skirt lengths should end above or below the knee, not on the knee. They don't have to be mini or micro-mini if they are above the knee. If below the knee, avoid lengths that cut across the widest part of your calf:

Pencil – a timeless shape that hugs the thigh and curves into the knee.

The 'A' line extends out from the hipline. This shape does not conceal bottom-heavy figures; it can create the illusion of looking bigger.

Full skirt - feminine and can be casual or formal.

Bias Cut – great for curves and always worn below the knee.

6. Style Basic Dresses

Some women find dresses easier because of the one-and-done factor, avoiding the pairing of top to bottom and the optional elimination of a waistband:

Body Con – a fitted dress of any length, neckline with sleeves or sleeveless.

Shift Dress—a looser fit than the Body Con, in lengths from micro-mini to below the knee, any neckline, sleeveless, or any sleeve style.

Shirt Dress – a shirt but longer, straight, full, patterned or plain.

Wrap Dress – below the knee, always a v-front, best tied high on the waist.

Skater Dress – a Body Con with a full skirt, short to midi length.

Maxi Dress – Full length, can be bias cut, gipsy style, flared, full, strappy, halter neck or with any style sleeve.

7. Style Basic Coats

Coats are often the first item to be seen and should be considered part of your overall style and look. Invest in your coats, or they will cover up your style:

Trench – travels through time, weather and seasons and can be any colour.

Winter Coat – ¾ to the knee is the most flattering, and stand-up collars allow for options with scarves and handbag straps.

Wraps & Capes - add drama and/or glamour, work through

seasons, work over chunky knits, and can be paired with longer gloves if cold wrists/arms are an issue.

2.3 Amend, Mend & Never Make-do

Amending clothes to fit your body and style can be as simple as taking up a trouser hem or as complex as reconstructing a jacket to change its style. *Mending* clothes, on the other hand, is replacing a broken zip, repairing a split seam or darning a moth hole to make loved garments last longer. Making do with clothes that don't quite fit you or your style or are beyond repair is not an option if you want your clothes to make you feel good and stylish. This section is designed to highlight some easy-to-fix problems in most wardrobes.

Firstly, never make do. If a garment does not fit your body, is not your style, is not appropriate for your current lifestyle or needs repair, then either do the necessary to amend or mend it or move it out of your wardrobe.

Garment alterations and repairs have an associated cost. Even if you are doing it yourself, it is time spent. Before you commit money or time, you must ensure that the alteration is worth the outcome.

To check, here are three questions:

1. Do you own better alternative garments that you reach for instead?
2. Do you love the garment enough to spend money on it?
3. Is the damage repairable or beyond repair?

Garment Repairs

Mending a garment that has accidental damage, such as a fabric tear, broken zip, detached button, or moth hole, is best done immediately so as not to disrupt your wardrobe flow.

I recall a client, Kelly, who had doggie treats in her coat pocket, and her eager pup jumped up and caught his tooth on the pocket, ripping the fabric clean away. This was her dog walking coat, an investment piece that was functional yet stylish and worn daily – she needed that fabric tear repaired pretty quickly if her wardrobe flow was not to be disrupted. (If the term 'wardrobe flow' sounds unfamiliar, it's because your wardrobe is not yet sorted into outfits – Chapter 5 will show you how).

Another way to decide if a repair is worth doing is to consider whether you feel the need to ask someone else's opinion. It's a regular occurrence for my clients to bring a bag of alterations to our sessions, and as they go through them, if they are humming and hawing about whether it's worth the spend, I always say 'no'; it can't be an integral piece of your wardrobe if you're not sure.

There are a few options when it comes to getting repairs done that you cannot do yourself:

1. You may already know someone, a relative, a local seamstress, or if not, start asking around.
2. Facebook is a great place as it has local search filters and recommendation options.
3. Most dry-cleaning shops offer garment repair and alteration services.
4. The sustainable living crisis has given rise to more garment repair and alteration services popping up everywhere. Even festivals or Earth Day celebrations have free 'repair shop' pop-ups.
5. There are online Apps like SOJO, which offer a collect-from-your-door service.
6. Or, if you are handy with a needle and thread and want to give it a go, YouTube can help with a variety of step-by-step instructional videos.

Whatever your option, don't wait—arrange your garment repairs as soon after the damage happens as possible.

Garment Alterations

There are two reasons why you would amend a garment: to alter its fit or to undertake what is known as a 're-fashion alteration'.

Fit alterations refer to things such as length adjustments, darts or seams taking in or letting out, and necklines reshaping. Fit alterations are usually done immediately after a garment is acquired, and some retail outlets offer an alterations service at the point of sale.

The same skills are required to undertake alterations and make repairs, so again, it is worth finding your local seamstress if you don't already know one. The cost associated with this type of amendment or alteration is usually a standard rate so if you feel the cost is too much to spend, then the question to ask is, do you need and love that garment? If you are unsure, the answer is probably a 'no'. (Worth vs Value will be covered next).

Fit alterations *can* happen after owning a garment for a while if, for example, the body shape changes. Also, fit alterations might be made if a garment is gifted in the wrong size or if pieces are handed down or are heirlooms. If the amendment is more complex than the standard alterations, be prepared for it to cost more.

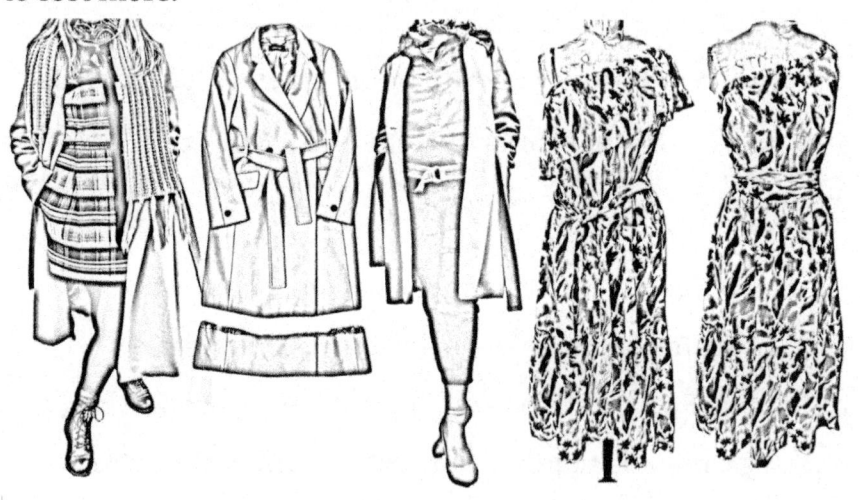

Wool Overcoat shortened & excess flounce removed from neckline

This long, tailored wool-mix coat was too formal for day-to-day styling and dressing it down was limited. Reducing the length by just 6" altered the overall outfit silhouette making it a versatile piece that can be worn with a multitude of outfits across all seasons.

The flounce around the neckline of this cotton print summer dress added bulk to a dress that was already voluminous. Removing the flounce-frill, accentuated the one-shoulder design, and the spare fabric was made into a wider belt to add a waist-shaping option.

A Re-fashion garment alteration involves separating and reconstructing a garment to alter the finished look. It takes more time and seamstress work, so it costs more. Re-fashioning can also be referred to as **Up-fashioning** or **Up-cycling**. Options here are endless and unique to each garment, allowing a complete transformation from the original into a bespoke piece. You will have full control of what you want to create, and it can be an excellent option for special occasions or for making sentimental pieces wearable. If you would like to know more about re-fashioning, refer to @myvosuk Instagram highlights or contact me via the website www.myvos.co.uk

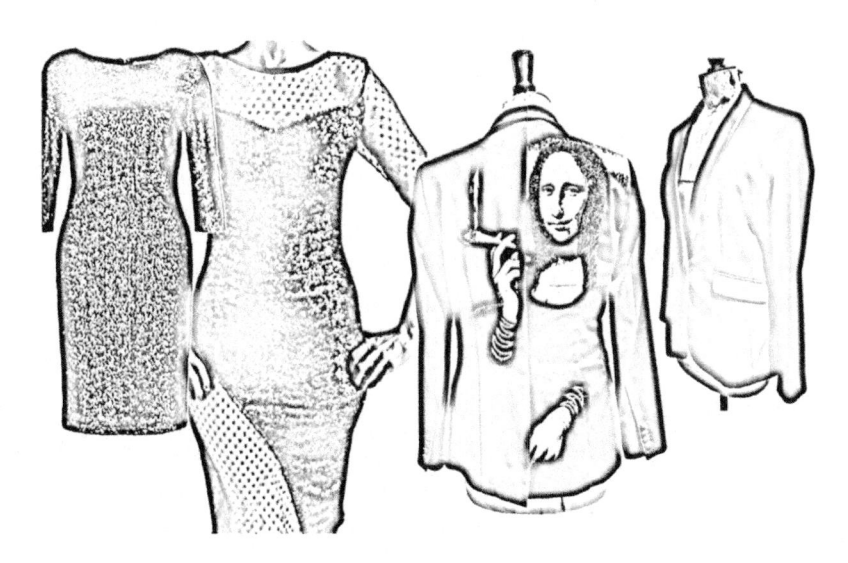

Re-fashioned Sequin dress adding length and contrasting sheer fabric.
Re-fashioned Tux. The back panel was created from an heirloom A-line skirt.

Amend, Mend And Never Make-Do - Summary

- Seamstress attention, whether it be repairs, minor alterations or complex re-fashions, comes at a cost. This should not outweigh the worth of a finished garment.
- Whether to undertake amendments should be carefully considered (for worth), and the outcome must be an item that fits you properly and aligns with your unique personal style (UPS).
- Alterations like hem or sleeve length amendments, fit adjustments on seams and darts, and neckline re-shaping should be carried out straight away, to make the garment instantly wearable. These are basic alterations that the seamstress can price up front for you.
- Repairs need to be made ASAP, too. If not, it suggests you no longer need or love the garment, or it has simply seen better days and is beyond repair.
- Never make-do. If a garment needs seamstress attention, amend, mend, or move it out of your wardrobe.
- Community repair shops are popping up as part of the wider sustainable future, so look out for them and use them.

Suggested Actions

1. Do you already use a seamstress or know where to get alterations done? If not, go back over the suggestions above to find out where you can get alterations done so you are prepared for when you do need them.
2. Do you currently have any garment repairs you can action now? If yes, don't wait, get them done.

3. If you would like more examples or information about garment re-fashioning go to @myvosuk Instagram highlights.

2.4 Worth, Value & Cost

The price tag of any garment, whether it is already hanging in your wardrobe or waiting to be purchased, has a different worth for everyone. So, when it comes to price, you only need to be concerned with what a garment is worth *to you*. Your lifestyle and budget will determine what money you spend; however, how each piece makes you feel ultimately decides its worth.

So, what determines the worth and value of your clothes?

It goes without saying that clothing purchases are based on budget and lifestyle preferences, however it's worth bearing in mind that price points can sway opinions (negatively) before full consideration has been given to the suitability, fit and style of the particular item. Though we all love a bargain, too many 'unsuitable' bargains will do nothing for your wardrobe except add chaos.

If you are questioning whether a garment or accessory is worth it before you decide to buy, then it could be that this item doesn't align with your needs. The fact that you are considering the purchase suggests you have the budget, so something else is holding you back from parting with your cash. Is it because you know it's not perfect but are short on time to look for anything else? I'll stop you there. Don't do it. **Make-do** is never an option when curating a stylish wardrobe. If you are happy to 'make-do', then wear something you already own and save today's budget for another time.

Cost Per Wear

Cost per wear is a calculation based on an item's purchase price divided by how often you are likely to wear it. In simple terms, if your new dress costs £30.00 and you will wear it once a month for a year, then the cost per wear for that item is 30 / 12 = £2.50 per wear.

If this formula worked, we would all be wearing expensive knickers and PJs and buying cheap Wedding dresses. I'm just kidding, but this concept has some credit if you add the value of how you feel, not just rely on maths.

For example, Jules was turning 40 and throwing a party to celebrate. She called upon my services to find the perfect dress to make her look the part and feel great. Her current wardrobe contained high-street brands like Zara and M&S, some Oliver Bonas, and a few reduced-sale items from Ted Baker. Jules told me she was willing to 'splurge', but I sensed her top price would be around the full, non-sale price of her existing Ted Baker pieces.

We found three nearly perfect dresses before deciding on the French Connection Body Con dress. This had a sheer layer of mesh heavily encrusted with sparkly sequins and beads that cascaded over the shoulders and graduated to a speck of sparkle at the hemline.

The problem, though, was the conservative neckline, which made it a tad formal. After further consideration, Jules and I agreed that a deep plunging V neckline would add sassiness to this classy number and create the perfect party vibe Jules wanted.

A decision was made, and I carried out the alteration. We added killer heels, a sparkly handbag, and an OTT sparkly statement necklace – pièce de résistance – perfect for her glitterball party.

The cost of hiring me plus the alteration meant Jules's dress spend was over budget, but we kept costs down by pairing it with shoes she already owned, and her friends clubbed together to buy the necklace and handbag as her 40th gift.

Since then, Jules has worn all the individual pieces in a multitude of outfit combinations, so not only did her one-off party look serve her well on the night, but every piece turned out to be a worthwhile investment that she still wears eight years on. A 'worth and value' jackpot.

Another client, Tania, messaged me to ask if £90 was worth it for a tweed percher (bespoke handmade headpiece) to complete her Race Day outfit. To me, it was a no-brainer; however, for Tania, who is not a regular Racegoer, there was no value to her or her wardrobe in owning this piece beyond that one day. Instead, I suggested she didn't part with her money and opt for a wide black velvet headband to complete her outfit. The headband looked striking against her freshly bleached, chopped bob hairstyle and complemented her black, knee-high boots. Tania got so much value from her headband choice that she purchased black velvet gloves and two more wide headbands. In the end, she spent more than £90, but the value added to her wardrobe and newfound love of wearing wide headbands elevated her look and the rest of her outfit combinations for the entire season, not just one day. Worth the spend.

Sticking To Budget

At times, we all go over budget because we see the worth of a garment. The investment over time, wearability, and feeling good add value to our look and wardrobe.

The two client examples are both occasion-related scenarios, and it is usually when we find ourselves in situations where we need to dress for something specific, rather than our daily routines, that we feel most vulnerable and emotional about our wardrobe and choice of clothing.

Other triggers come when we encounter new people and notice they look good, causing us to check if we look good, too.

When it comes to budget, spend according to your gut feeling. This is the best way to check the worth and value of every item you buy. If you are shopping simply for the pleasure of the experience or are selecting the best out of a bad bunch, you will have neither worth nor valued pieces.

Low To High Price-Tags

Worth in monetary terms alone will not make you stylish. Just because a piece is expensive doesn't automatically make it your style.

The cheapest new clothing is found in supermarkets, large stores like Matalan, and high-street shops like Primark. These companies have hundreds of stores as well as e-commerce outlets and sell tens of thousands of any one design across a wide range of sizes. Cost is kept affordable by using low-cost fabrics and the cheapest production methods, all of which fall into the 'fast fashion' bracket we discussed earlier. Other online marketplaces have grown recently, with names such as Shein and Temu lowering clothing prices even further.

High-end pieces are the opposite. These are made from premium materials and are produced in limited quantities and sizes. They also have the highest standards of finishing detail and are associated with prestigious fashion houses. High-end pieces will be 'papped' being worn by the rich and famous which means you are also paying for the privilege of joining the fashion elite within the price tag.

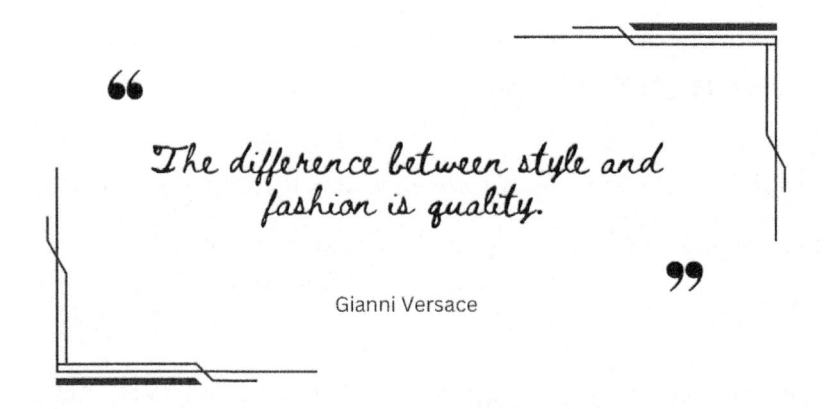

> *The difference between style and fashion is quality.*
>
> Gianni Versace

Between these two extremes is the middle ground, a sliding scale of affordability between low and high-priced garments weighed up against value and worth. The consideration here is often deciding if what you are getting with the higher-priced garment is worth the same value as what you are losing with the cheaper-priced garment.

There are two major players in this middle ground—the ethical and the pre-loved markets. Both dramatically reduce the consumer's clothing costs but in very different ways. The pre-loved market has advanced from being referred to as items 'discreetly disposed' in the 1920s to what is now the hottest growing trend of the 21st century. We're going to talk about pre-loved a bit more later.

Sustainable Clothing

When it comes to the ethical market, there is a huge amount to consider. Beneath the surface of a garment price tag is a much more complex, sinister side which we need to fully understand in order to embrace the true monetary value of an item. The price alone does not (always) provide an accurate representation of its cost – here's why:

1. The exponential growth of low-price fast fashion, and more recently ultra-fast fashion, has been made possible by the use of cheaper fabrics – but that's not all. Sadly, this shift has come at a considerable cost to workers in the textile industry and has caused an incredible amount of damage to our planet.
2. The exploitation of people, mainly but not exclusively in developing countries, coupled with major environmental factors surrounding pollution and CO2 emissions, are significant contributors to low-price clothing.
3. There is a belief I hear a lot, a statement really, which says that if the garment has already been made, then the damage (to the workforce and environment) has already been done, so there is no harm in purchasing it. To an extent, there is truth in this argument, but this is CRITICAL; **only when we stop buying will the demand be reduced. And only then will the exploitation of workers and environmental damage slow down.**

To put sustainability into context, here are some statistics, as reported on www.earth.org:

- 100 billion garments are produced each year.
- Of which, 92 million tonnes end up in landfills, the equivalent of a rubbish truck full of clothes dumped in

- landfill sites every second.
- The fashion industry is responsible for 20% of global wastewater.
- Nearly 10% of microplastics dispersed in the ocean each year come from textiles.
- 16 million tonnes of CO2 emissions were created in the US in 2020 from returned purchases alone.

So, it isn't just buying the clothes, it is the way we are disposing of them, too.

Clothes we buy or acquire on a 'make-do' basis or pick up from the bargain bucket are typically the ones we don't value and are the easiest to get rid of. If a garment only has a 'one-time wear' value to you (and/or has minimal monetary worth), it will almost certainly end up in a landfill site.

Martina Igini's article, '10 Concerning Fast Fashion Waste Statistics', which you can also find on www,earth.org suggests that the apparel industry's global emissions will increase by 50% in less than seven years **unless** we stop buying fast fashion.

This is the only way we can reduce demand and slow down the effects of production, and, in doing so, champion slow rather than fast fashion.

There is good news, though. Pre-loved is the hottest growing trend, and stores like TK Maxx are making quality garments affordable, dramatically reducing the production and waste cycle damaging the planet.

This is what TK Maxx says about its customers,

> *"Our buyers are opportunistic and entrepreneurial. So when a designer overproduces, or other stores overbuy, we swoop in, negotiate the lowest possible price and pass the savings on."*

If your current habits and budget are in the fast fashion category, you will understandably be concerned about the affordability of clothing that is not fast fashion, but there are options available to meet both the desire to shop and keep a cap on your clothing spend. When worth and value become an integral part of your clothing decision-making process, your style will automatically elevate, too.

In simple terms, it's about quality over quantity—but it's even more than that. It's about having the right items in your wardrobe so that you can reduce spending and waste without forgoing style, functionality, and wearability.

We're going to cover more about shopping options in Chapter 7.

Worth, Value And Cost - Summary

- Worth and value should not be viewed as either or. The cost attached to clothing goes deeper than the price tag and requires you to establish your truth and ethics towards the worth and value of your clothes collection, as well as future purchases.
- The production and expiration of cheap clothes is not sustainable and comes at a high cost to the planet and exploitation of the textile workforce.
- The pre-loved market provides options to buy at a higher price, knowing that it has a re-sell value to add to your budget.
- A stylish wardrobe that brings joy will have a mix of items from varying price points because it's not the price tag that determines if a piece is perfect for you.

Suggested Actions

Price ranging will help determine where to shop and source future items.

Clothing Budget

ITEM	PRICE
Overcoat	£ -£
Jacket	£ -£
Sweater/Sweatshirt	£ -£
Blouse/Shirt	£ -£
Trousers	£ -£
Dress/Jumpsuit	£ -£
Skirt	£ -£
Vest/Cami	£ -£
Footwear	£ -£
Handbags	£ -£
....	£ -£
....	£ -£
....	£ -£
....	£ -£
....	£ -£

Further Reading – Environment & Sustainability

As I've alluded to, sustainability is a huge topic in the clothing industry, and there are many articles written by journalists, bloggers, activists, bbc.com and Gov.org that explain the consequences of excess clothing production and provide guidance on how to reduce it. I definitely recommend further reading and have included a few links below:

1. Earth.org provides up-to-date statistics with future predictions if changes are not made.
   - earth.org/fast-fashions-detrimental-effect-on-the-environment/
   - earth.org/statistics-about-fast-fashion-waste/
   - bbc.com/future/article/20200310-sustainable-fashion-how-to-buy-clothes-good-for-the-climate/

2. Goodonyou.eco provides daily advice on all things clothing and planet friendly. You can sign up to their mailing list for information on things like eco brand recommendations, and garment longevity tips.

In an interview for the Guardian June 2023, Mary Portas said,

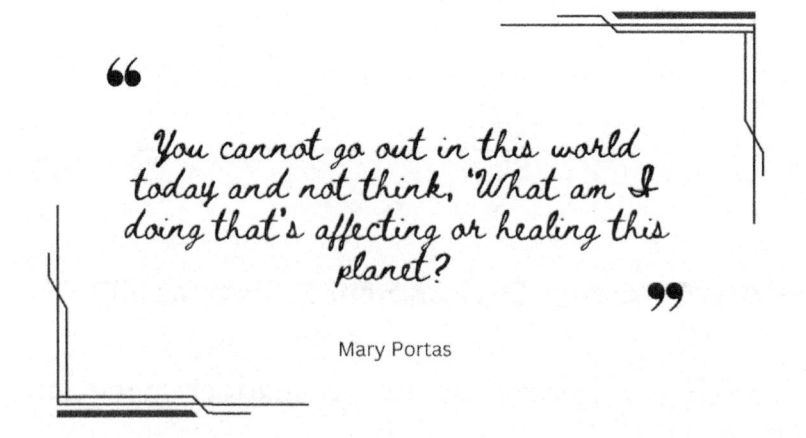

> *You cannot go out in this world today and not think, "What am I doing that's affecting or healing this planet?"*
>
> Mary Portas

125

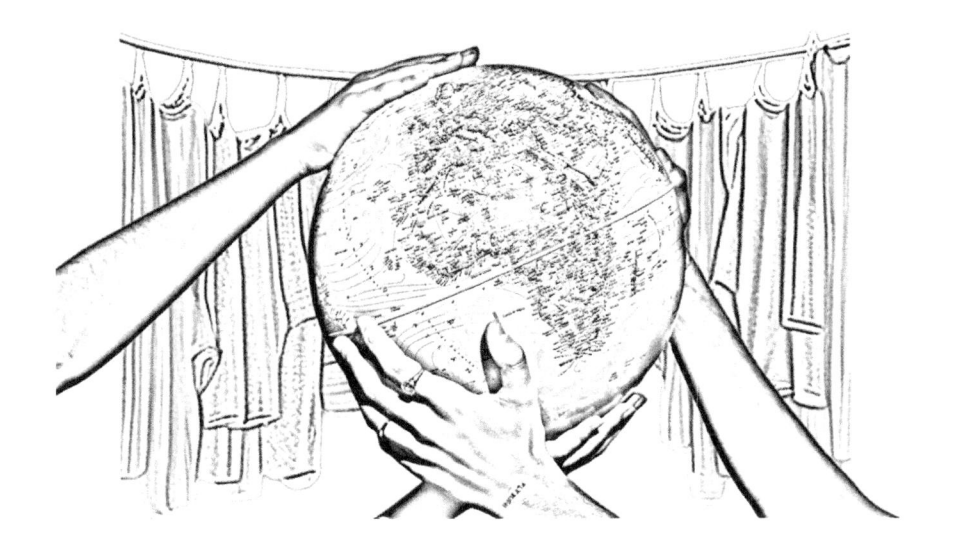

3. Style Formulas

In previous chapters, we've examined style and how we can begin to dress and select our clothes based on the style that works best for us. However, we can also use the principle of a formula to help. Many style formulas use a sequence to help how we dress, and these can be adapted when required.

When To Use A Style Formula

The ideal time to employ a style formula is when you feel stuck with what to wear, are bored with your current collection, or fancy an enjoyable style boost.

If your wardrobe is in a muddle and more of your clothes feel like 'make-do' items rather than beloved garments, then a style formula can provide a structured, focused re-start and give you the direction needed to get back on track. Even the most stylish, confident dressers become bored with their wardrobes and crave an injection of style excitement.

Most style formulas involve a one-to-one get-together with a stylist. This could take place in your home or perhaps at their studio and doesn't necessarily need to be a formal affair. Some stylists offer services as group workshops or as parties for groups of friends. Whether a gift, a treat, or a dose of TLC, style-boosting formulas can be fun as well as informative.

You may also want to seek the help of a style formula if you have:
1. A diverse collection of individual garments that don't form outfits easily.
2. The habit of wearing the same outfits on rotation.
3. A tendency to 'repeat-buy' clothes.

Or you might be someone who:
1. Doesn't have much of an interest in clothes or shopping

for clothes.
2. Has already spent time experimenting with colours and styles to no avail.
3. Doesn't feel confident and would like some expert help.

All of these are great reasons to consider using a style formula.

What Are The Style Formulas

The three most popular style formulas are:

1. Personal Colour Analysis

2. Style Personality Testing

3. How to Dress Your Body Shape

Each formula has pros and cons regarding its effectiveness, but regardless of their individual outcome, they are all enjoyable experiences.

Let's investigate.

> ...clothing is a form of self-expression. There are hints about who you are in what you wear.
>
> Marc Jacobs

3.1 Personal Colour Analysis

Have you ever put something on and thought that the colour washed you out? Or perhaps you noticed someone wearing a colour, and all you saw was the colour rather than the person?

Did you know everyone can wear any colour if it's the right shade?

Well, they can. Welcome to the world of colour and clothing.

Personal Colour Analysis is a method of finding out which colours look best on you, with the intention of helping you choose clothes in colours that suit you. It is carried out by a trained Colour Consultant, who is also likely to be a personal stylist or hair stylist.

The theory is to complement your natural colouring, which

includes your skin shade, eye shade, and lip colour. It might not sound exciting, but it is genuinely fascinating!

The clarity of colours tested takes into account whether you are:

1. Cool or Warm – warm palettes contain yellow, whilst cool palettes have a hint of blue.
2. Deep or Light - the darkest to lightest shades that suit you.
3. Clear or Soft - the brightest shade of colour to the most muted.

The Colour Consultant will sit you in a well-lit area and ask you to remove any make-up. You will then be given a white, salon-like robe to cover your shoulders and a white hairband to cover your hairline. This all takes place in front of a mirror.

At this point, the reflection in the mirror is probably not your best (!), but the consultant will then begin draping a myriad of coloured cloths under your chin to cover your decolletage. The light then reflects the colour from your chest to your face, and you can compare the different colours.

The process will also identify colours that emphasise under-eye bags and deeper wrinkle lines or those that highlight skin blemishes you incessantly try to disguise.

There's more. Some colours can make your thinning lips

disappear or blend so well with your skin that they give the illusion of dragging your face downwards, causing your jowls to form a double chin! Whilst those might not sound like fun discoveries, I've yet to meet anyone who hasn't found the overall experience fascinating and hugely enjoyable. Remember, though, colour is just one part of the formula and is certainly not the entire solution to dressing well forever.

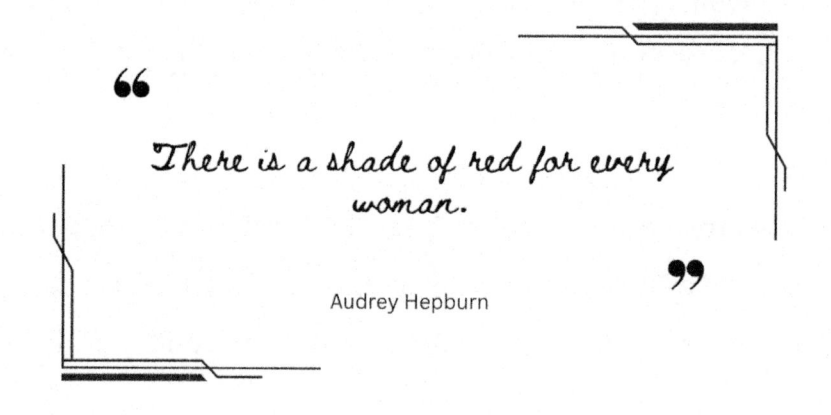

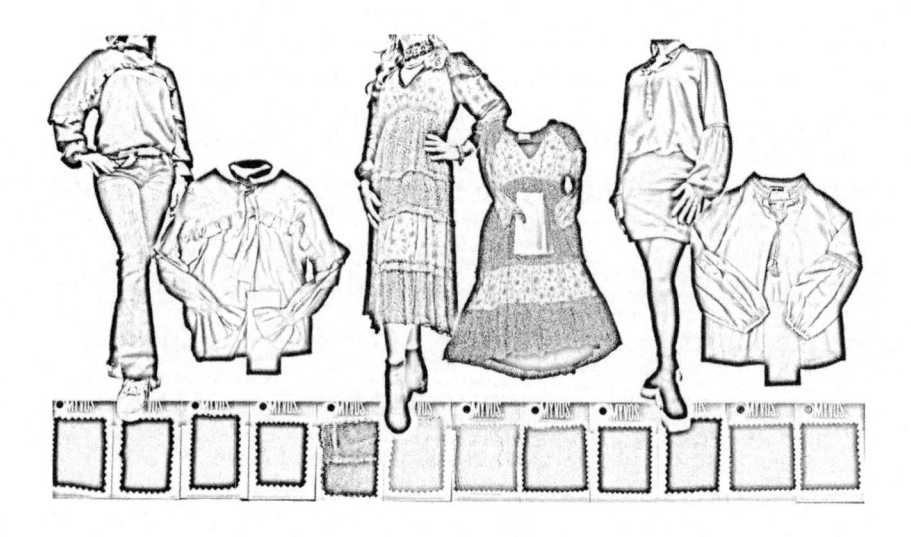

> *There is a shade of red for every woman.*
>
> Audrey Hepburn

When Colour Is Overused

If you consistently wear the same colour to the point it is the most prominent part of your look, it will become more representative of a Uniform than a personal style. Whilst uniforms are a form of recognition and trust, this look does not translate well to an individual's personal style. Avoid this by making sure that your wardrobe and choice are not restricted to one colour only.

At the end of your Colour Analysis Consultation, you will be given a swatch wallet containing your best colours. This is for you to keep and should comprise a selection of neutral colours, base colours, and additional trend colours, with advice on how to wear them.

The consultation should also cover an idea of how to implement your new colours into your existing wardrobe and future purchases. I have met women who purchase a scarf or cardigan in their 'best' advised colour at the end of their consultation, often selected from the Colour Consultant's current stock. Sometimes, they will also purchase a matching lipstick and leave happy, thinking they have what they need to add a pop of colour to any outfit. This look may well work for a few outfits, but it will become dated and formulaic if you're not careful. The scarf/cardigan/lipstick is part of your outfit, including attention to silhouette, proportion, fabric and fit. As I've said above – stylish dressing is not just about colour.

If you want to create a dramatic personal style, you can use the reverse of your colour analysis. One of the questions I posed earlier was whether you'd ever seen someone and commented that the 'dress was wearing them' rather than the other way around. This is what you can create – if you wish to – by using the reverse of your optimal colours. Stage performers use colour to look conspicuous to a large crowd on stage, so if you are going somewhere special and want to make an impact or an entrance, going bold on a colour that is not in your harmonious palette can do this. We are going to talk more about developing style in Chapter 7.

Colour Analysis Pros

- Introduce you to new colour options that harmonise with your natural colouring.
- Use the illusion of colour to accentuate body shape.
- Reduce and declutter a large assortment of clothes.
- Confirm the colours you are wearing are the best ones for you.
- Confidently add colour to a mostly neutral clothes collection.
- Define colours that can be worn for a momentous

occasion.
- Have an uplifting experience individually or with friends.

Colour Analysis Cons

- A colour formula is part of personal style, not the only element.
- One colour can become a uniform look rather than a stylish look.
- Colour is assessed next to your skin in daylight. Results are less noticeable on garments away from the face and hands, or in dark lighting.
- Re-assessment of colours is recommended when signs of natural colouring change—for example, greying hair.
- Personal style upstages colour - clothing choices made solely on colour can look dated.

Capsule Collections

Capsule Collections consist of a limited number of items that work together to create many outfit options. They are a great concept when wardrobe space is limited, when travelling, or when creating a 'business' wardrobe.

Capsules are also useful for periods in life that are not permanent, for example, temporary employment or contract work, a change of lifestyle role, or a body shape change due to medication or illness that will not be permanent.

Clothing choices based around a limited palette of complimentary colours offers the best way to create a capsule collection.

Personal Colour Analysis - Summary

- Personal Colour Analysis tests what colours compliment the natural colouring of your skin, eyes and lips.
- The process is fun, informative, fascinating and an enjoyable experience.
- Colour is also used in outfit formulas to give figure shaping illusions, such as matching to bottom colour will elongate and look taller, or lighter colour on top and darker on the bottom will widen shoulders and narrow hips.

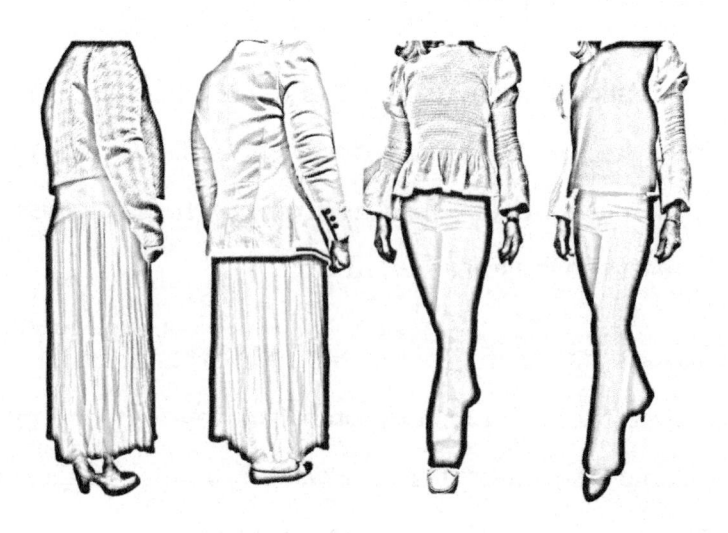

5'5" Size14 | 5'2" Size06

The same Colour top and bottom creates the illusion of height.
Lighter Colour on the top creates the illusion of
wider shoulders and narrower hips.

> I love bright colours whatever the season particularly 'jewelled colours.' I feel different when I wear colour. I feel in my happy place.
>
> Julia, Education and Business Ambassador

3.2 Dress your Shape

We have touched upon the five typically used formulaic body shapes in *Chapter 1.4 – Body Beautiful Before Clothes*. **Dress Your Shape** formulas use these five body form categories to identify your body shape and follow a corresponding list of suggested clothing shapes to match.

The Dress Your Shape Consultant will provide accompanying annotations and descriptions of how each garment style suggestion accentuates, conceals, or balances your body. A shopping trip is usually part of the package deal.

Here is how the figures of our ladies from Chapter 1 translate into formulaic body shapes.

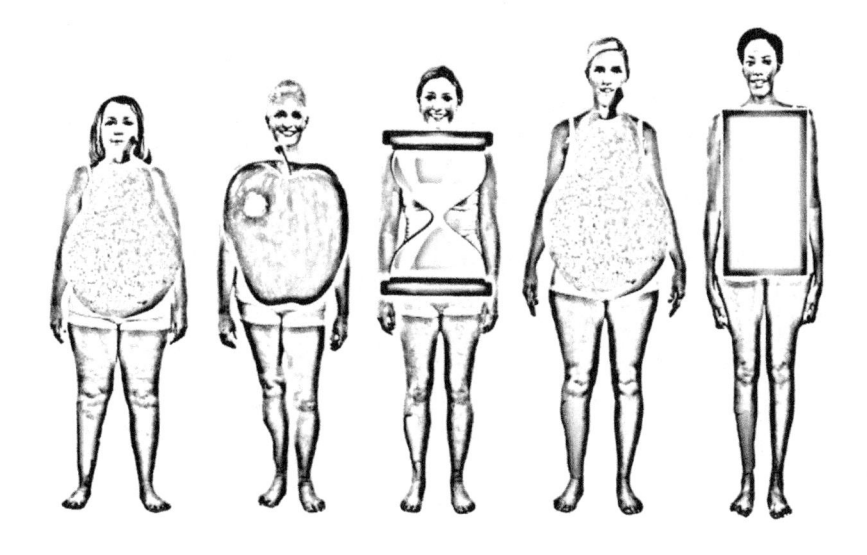

5'2" Size14 | 5'4" Size18 | 5'8" Size12 | 5'11" Size12 | 6'1" Size10

Body shapes translated into formulaic shapes
From Left to Right - Hourglass, Pear, Apple, Inverted Triangle, Rectangle

Dress Your Shape Pros

1. The formula will be helpful if you are one of these shapes with an average bust size.
2. Increases confidence to go shopping and experiment with trying clothes on.
3. It gets you looking at your body shape and trying on clothes you would typically avoid.
4. It is a positive experience to work with a consultant who will teach you tips on how to accentuate or disguise body areas.

Dress Your Shape Cons

1. Body shape includes height, not just shoulder, waist, and hip proportions, so it's not foolproof if these aren't considered during your Consultation.
2. Body proportions such as short in the body and long legs, or long in the body and short legs, etc, change the overall outfit silhouette, so again, these need to be considered.
3. Side and back angles and front view body shape need to be considered.
4. Bust size variations, small or large, add another variant to apple, pear and rectangle shapes.

Here are the suggestions if you do fall into a defined formula shape category:

Body Shape Tips

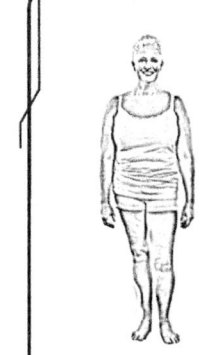

Smaller on the bottom:
Choose drapey fabrics on top & stiff/rigid fabrics on bottom.

Jumpsuits work well.

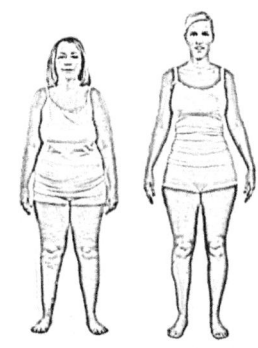

Smaller on top:
Drapey fabrics on the bottom, with a little stretch & any fabric on top.

Bias cut skirts work well.

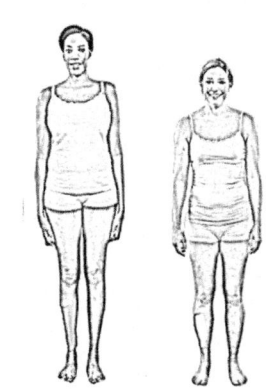

Equal Shoulder/Hip:
Your height and curvature will termine best fabrics, cuts & styles.

Dresses work well.

Dress Your Shape – Summary

- Trying clothes on and looking in the mirror is often a more effective and efficient way of seeing what suits you, especially as your body naturally succumbs to shape change over time.
- As explained in Chapter 2, fabric variants and fit alter your overall dressed silhouette.
- Consuming time analysing an inch here or there to work out if your hips are wider than your shoulders or if an expanding waistline is considered an hourglass is not the most efficient way to be stylish.
- You will already have an idea of what suits your shape, so have the confidence to continually try on and test a variety of garments. Then, you will reap the biggest rewards.

> "I think whatever size or shape body you have, it's important to embrace it and get down!"
>
> Christina Aguilera

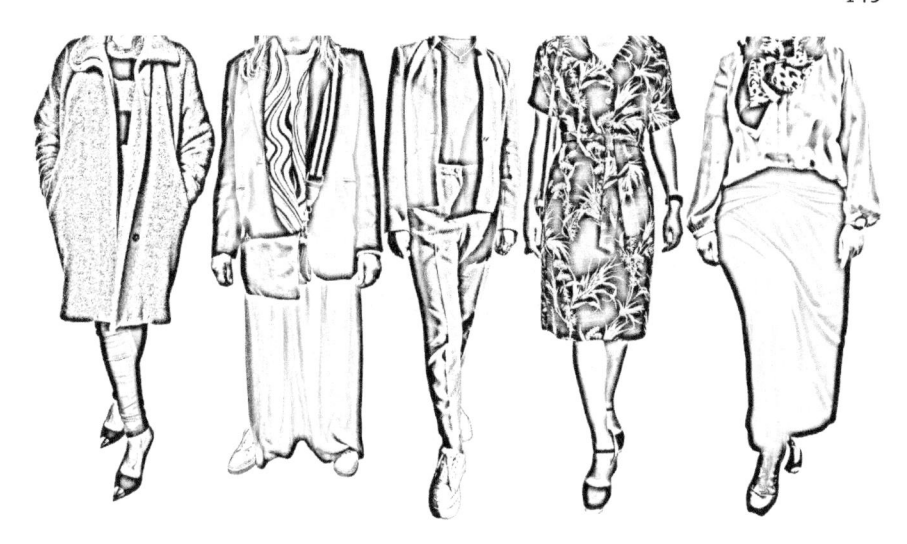

5'2" Size14 | 5'4" Size16 | 5'6" Size08 | 5'5" Size10 | 5'5" Size18
Left to Right: Smaller on Bottom, Smaller on Bottom, Same, Same, Smaller on Top

Wear your gorgeous clothes, rather than thinking about fruit shapes!

3.3 Style Personality Formula

A style personality can be described as *'how the traits of your personality and character are communicated through your clothing'*.

Using the formula route to decipher your style personality usually starts with a multiple-choice questionnaire. These questionnaires vary in length and can be completed independently or as part of a style consultation. Your answers will be totalled to reveal your 'style personality' type. There are typically six categories of style personality:

1. Classic or Minimalist
2. Creative or Arty
3. Natural or Relaxed
4. Dramatic or Magnetic
5. Polished or City Chic
6. Romantic or Bohemian

Depending on where you are in the world or whose questionnaire you complete, the types will vary. I don't tend to use 'polished' as a style personality category because, in my opinion, all categories, even casual and natural styles, need to be 'polished' to be stylish.

Each category is coupled with visuals of an iconic celebrity to clarify the differences between style categories. Here are a few examples:

- Classic = Audrey Hepburn
- Chic = Jackie O
- Natural= Kate Winslet
- Romantic = Sarah Jessica Parker

As with the previous two formulas, not everyone will fall neatly into one category. For example, Naturals can be Natural-Classic or Natural-Creative, Classics can be Classic-Magnetic or Classic-Chic, and the variables go on. You can find your current style personality by selecting the best 5%-15% of your existing clothes collection – the clothes you love the very most, regardless of whether you currently wear them - and then identify your own theme to describe them. Are they textured, patterned, flowered, plain, detailed, formal, relaxed, bohemian, colourful, floaty, fitted... (you can use any of the descriptive words and categories already mentioned too.)

This reverse method of starting with your favourite clothes skips the need for a questionnaire and prevents you from trying to shoe-horn yourself into a category that you feel is 'nearest' to you rather than the 'real' you.

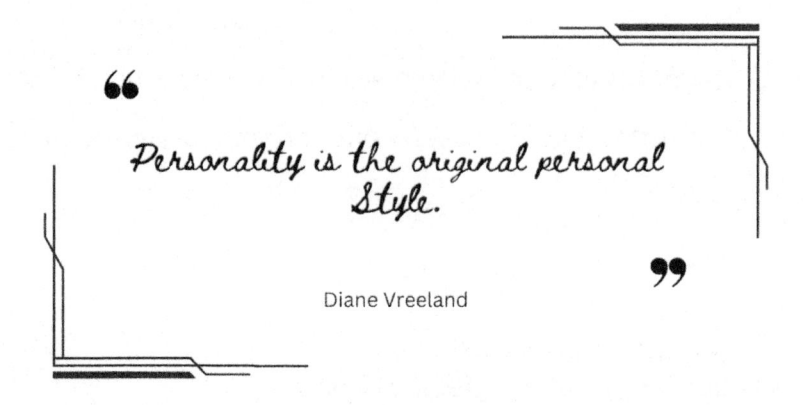

> *Personality is the original personal style.*
>
> — Diane Vreeland

Style Personality Pros

1. A great starting point if you need a confidence boost.
2. Gets you thinking and acknowledging your favourite clothes.
3. A positive experience to work with an Image Consultant who will encourage you to wear your best.

Style Personality Cons

1. Your unique personal style (UPS) may not fit into a formulaic category.
2. Focusing on one 'Style Type' category may not align

with every aspect of your lifestyle.
3. Can conflict with creating a signature look.

Style Personality - Summary

- Taking a style personality quiz can be great fun and a good starting point if you have no idea how to define your style or clothes. However, you are unlikely to slot perfectly into one category.
- We have already established that 'make-do' is not an option when it comes to being stylish forever, and that includes *not making do* with a category just because it's on a list. (We will discuss defining your UPS in the next few chapters).
- My style personality is Romantic, and my dominant colour palette is Soft. These two pieces of information alone will not serve me well – I have yet to see a Romantic section in a shop and if there was, would the garments on offer be my cut, proportion, fit, and in a Soft colour palette? Nope. Because a standalone formula is an *enjoyable confidence-boost*, but it only makes up part of your style choices and is *not a forever style fix*.

Suggested Actions

Make some notes about your thoughts towards Style Formulas and how they have/have not helped you:

1. What Style formulas have you done?
2. When did you have them done?
3. How did they help you dress?
4. Are you considering using a style formula?

5. How do you think it will help you with your clothing choices and style?

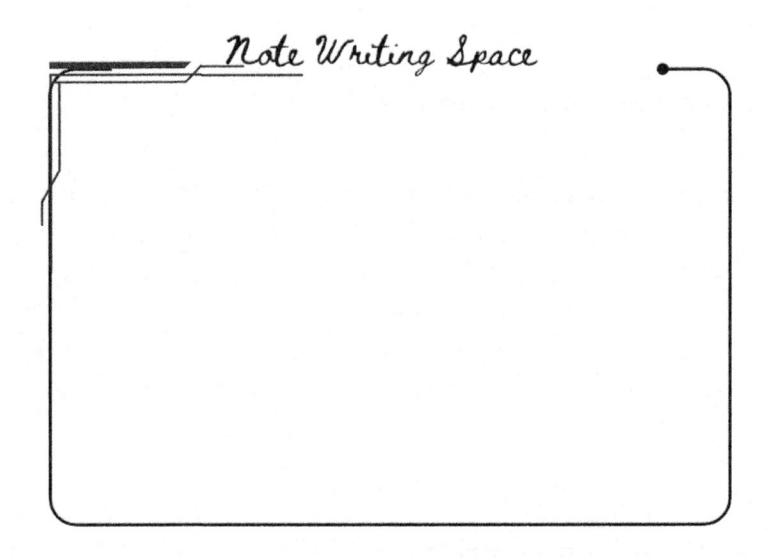

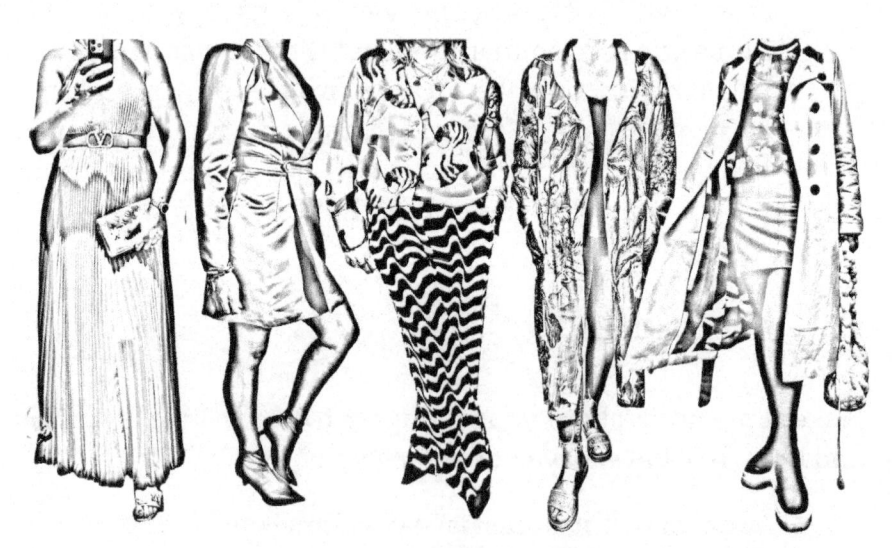

Note Writing Space

5'11" Size14 | 5'0" Size08 | 5'2" Size14 | 5'9" Size16 | 5'6" Size12

Style Personalities is having the confidence to wear what you love. Style Personalities is having the confidence to wear what you love.

4. Daily Dress Code

"I'm not going anywhere special, so it doesn't matter what I wear."

I hear this often, quickly followed by, "What shall I wear? Does it matter or not?"

The answer is yes; it does matter because getting dressed is a two-way visual—what you are presenting and what others see.

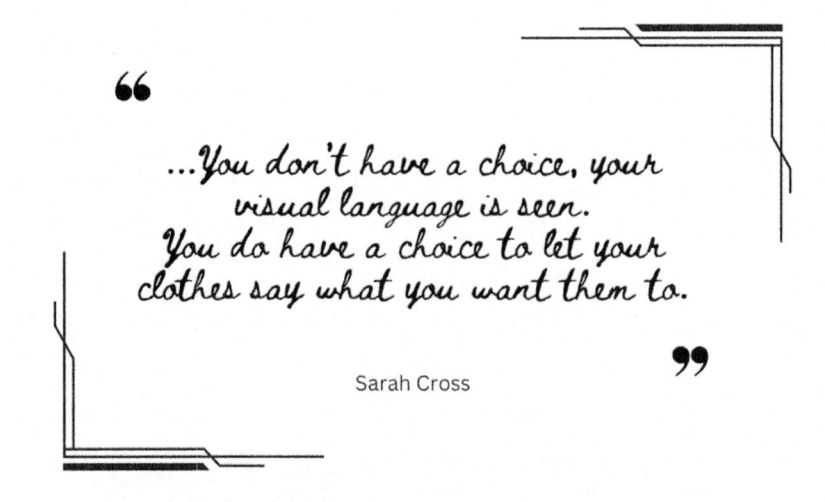

> *...You don't have a choice, your visual language is seen. You do have a choice to let your clothes say what you want them to.*
>
> — Sarah Cross

If you don't bother to take a step back, look in the mirror, and asses what *you* look like, that doesn't mean nobody will notice. Others will still look, and *they* will determine your style category.

Anna is 45 years old, and her 'jeans and jumper look' was described as 'Mumsie'. She is a mother to daughter Alex, now 19, who is away at university. However, the label given to Anna by her peers really touched a nerve. She revelled in being Mumsie when Alex was a baby, but nearly two decades later, the label made her feel frumpy, characterless, and even invisible.

Another client, Judi, wears jeans and jumpers, too. Her style is natural, elegant, and effortless. Her UPS has a hint of creativity. Her jeans are frayed at the hems, short enough to expose her pumps' silver-grey leather ankle strap and hem width, equalling her thigh-width, so her legs look elongated. She paired it with a thin, soft grey sweater that hung slightly longer at the back and followed the same line as her untucked shirt tails, which showed 1cm below her jumper. Judi accessorises with just one piece of oversized statement jewellery – a ring *or* large earrings, colourful and glazed-like art pieces. She loves a scarf, too. Floaty in the summer season and more of a wrap-around her shoulders in the cooler months – not the same wrap year-on-year either. She includes a surprise poncho or tailored waistcoat in soft, muted colours like her sweater collection. Judi's styling of jeans and sweaters showcased her attention to detail, silhouette, fabrics, and personal love of bright colours that appeared in just a hint within her jewellery.

Anna's 'Mumsie' look, which also included jeans and jumpers, did not showcase any attention to silhouette, cut of trouser leg, or footwear. With no accessories or focal point to her outfit, it was obvious that her random jumpers were not flattering to her shape.

Like any Visual Language, everything is there for a reason. In this chapter, you will learn how to find your levels of dress code, adapt your dress codes to align with your daily dressing, and how to inject your UPS.

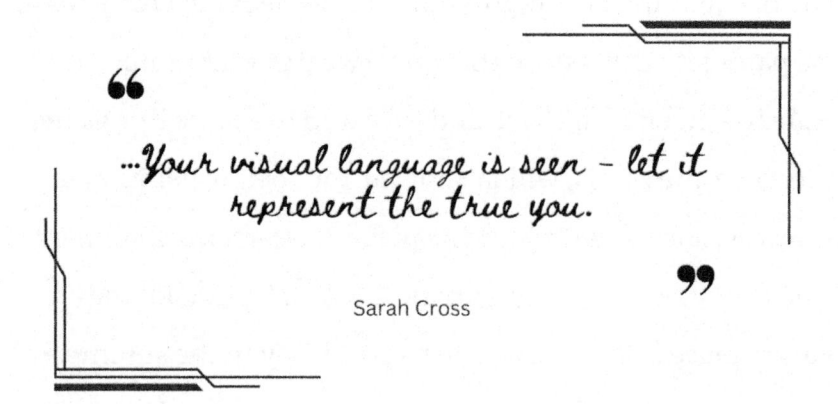

> *...Your visual language is seen – let it represent the true you.*
>
> Sarah Cross

4.1 The 5 Levels of Dress Code

The *dress code* refers to an expected standard of what to wear. For most, it is associated with weddings, Black Tie events, club entry, and work, the sorts of events that are specific occasions or scenarios you would expect to have a code of conduct for.

The 5 Levels of Dress Code methods you will learn here are different in that they will form your daily dressing boundaries to match and align with your specific lifestyle. It starts from level 1, which is your most casual jimjams, and goes up to level 5, which is your most formal, dressy attire. The middle level - level 3, is your daily 'go-to' attire. So, how does level dressing work?

Applying a dress code to your daily dressing habits provides an easy strategy when it comes to knowing what to wear for any given situation. You will be prepared in advance for whether you need to dress up or dress down, so when there is a change, you're ready for it without the heart-sinking feeling of wondering what to wear. Plus, you will already know your outfit feels like you, giving you more confidence before facing a situation that is not necessarily your daily routine.

Marcia, who I met at a business network group, was worried about what to wear to an upcoming board meeting. A year ago, she left her employment to set up her independent mortgage consultancy, and her new daily routine was WFH. This shifted her towards the more relaxed attire we adopted after the world pandemic, meaning her dress code had changed from formal suits and heels to casual with no thought about shoes. Marcia no longer knew how to dress for a board meeting. Her WFH casuals were not boardroom attire, yet returning to her suits and court shoes didn't feel right either. I suggested one of the smart-casual dresses I had seen her in at network meetings, paired with a nude, closed-toe, block-heel shoe to replace her somewhat scruffy black trainers. I also suggested adding a third piece, such as a soft, tailored, short-fitted jacket in a plain colour.

Replacing Marcia's relaxed black trainers with a nude shoe and adding the soft tailored jacket easily took her daily dress code up a level. Both pieces, shoes and jacket, could be paired with most of Marcia's daily go-to clothes to dress them up a level at any time, eliminating the worry of what to wear when she was expected at a meeting.

Each level of the daily dress code does a different job and represents a shift in formality, although all levels form part of your complete clothes collection. You will see when we look at the levels in a bit more detail that Level 3 is your base look and accounts for the largest part of what you dress for. You then have two levels up and two levels down. The more you use and implement this 5-level system, the more you will realise that you own lots of core garments which are suitable across several levels of your dress code. How you style the finished outfit, albeit as simple as a change of footwear or adding a more formal top layer, will differentiate between the levels.

Your clothes choices and overall look will follow a coherent style, and you will gain confidence just by opening your wardrobe door, knowing that 'what to wear' is not an issue.

I'm going to use my earth and environment analogy to explain the purpose of each of the five levels of dress code:

Level 1—Earth's Core and never seen.
This is your relaxed, at-home nightwear. Your private comfies, hidden away from outside eyes, are also worn when unwell and became popular in

the depths of lockdown.

Level 2 – Earth's Surface that adapts to climate and reacts to what is happening on land.

This is your first step up from being unseen to being seen. The level of dress code required as you go about your chores or are open to visitors. For example, popping to the gym, walking the dog, answering the door to a delivery driver, checking in on a neighbour, and even relaxing on a retreat holiday rather than at home. Level 2 exposes you to observers and comes with considerations of weather and functionality. It became a novelty norm for WFH newbies but has since become a mood-reducing level of dress code when worn daily.

Level 3 – Your base on Earth.

This dress code is the bulk of what you wear according to your daily life routine and the environment in which you live. This could be going to work, WFH, the school run, grocery shopping, meeting colleagues/friends, visiting family friends, caring for relatives, commuting, travelling… your day-to-day life dressing, in full view of observers, showcasing your visual language, expressing your values and tastes to the World.

Lifestyles that have minimal interaction with others, including WFH, often remain in the Level 2 dress code. As mentioned above, the Level 2 dress code is not all that good for wellbeing. It forms a habit that makes it overwhelming to dress for Level 4 and 5 occasions and can trigger the snowball effect of losing your style identity as well as confusion around what to wear. Get dressed in your Level 3 dress code even if you WFH or think you are unlikely to see anyone today.

Level 4 – Going to town.

You know you are stepping out somewhere where people will see you and make an internal judgement on how you present yourself, and you want it to be a good judgement. This is true of all Levels of Dressing;

however, Level 4 dressing matters to *you* more than *who's watching* because it is used when *you are dressing for what you want in life*. Including pitching to new clients, enjoying evenings out, going on a first date, an interview, attending social occasions and anniversaries, supporting your partner at a work-do, seeing your child collect an award, and all the occasions you feel needed. It is an upgrade on Level 3 that is necessary to feel good and confident and evolve in all aspects of your life.

Level 5 – The Big City Lights.

Your top level of dress code is for when there is no hiding. You will be seen, and an expectation will be put on you. It's your party, your promotion, your achievement, and you have the confidence to look the part, feel the part, and dress for it. Or you have an invite to celebrate someone else's big thing and the invite will set out the expected dress code.

The 5 Levels of Dress Code - example

5 Levels of Dress Code

5	Top Occasion	Dressy Celebrations, High-End Events, CEO Presentations etc.
4	Dress Up	Formal Events, Evening Wear, Interviews, Occasional Wear etc.
3	Base Level	Daily Dress, Work Wear, Uniform, Office Attire, Every Day Wear etc.
2	Dress Down	Leisure Wear, Weekend Attire, Holiday Clothes, Activewear etc.
1	Lounge Wear	Sleep Wear, Nightwear, and Loungewear.

> Knowing your Level 3 Dress Code is the key to knowing which of your garments fit into which level.

Your base Level 3 is your starting point and is determined by how you dress according to your daily lifestyle routine. For example, a financial advisor would be more formally dressed in the workplace than a landscape gardener. This does not make any difference to your five levels of dress code; it just means that your base level is of similar formality to the next level up or down but for different reasons. As mentioned, there are plenty of cases where individual garments cross over into several levels - the differentiation is how they are styled into outfit combinations. This is precisely what you aim for to achieve a coherent personal style, where you are always stylish whatever the occasion.

Aligning your clothes with what you are dressing for by recognising your different levels of formality or casualness makes it much easier to manage your wardrobe. It's more than owning a tidy wardrobe; it is an integral part of being able to dress stylishly and with ease and use your clothes to elevate your mood and well-being.

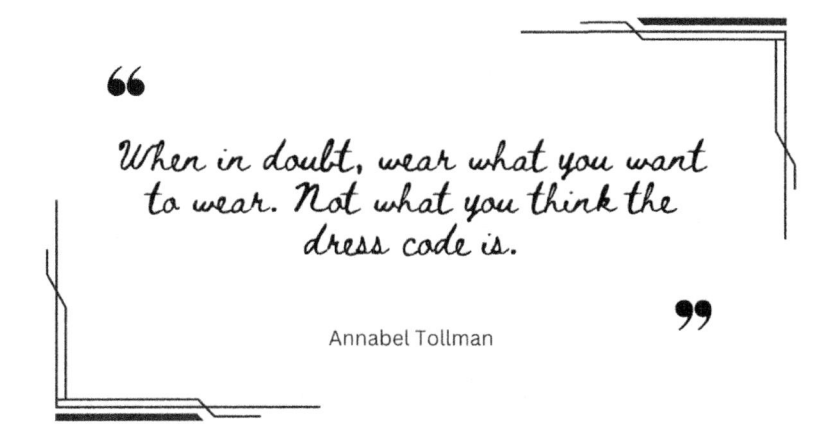

> *When in doubt, wear what you want to wear. Not what you think the dress code is.*
>
> Annabel Tollman

The 5 Levels Of Dress Code - Summary

- The 5 Levels of Dress Code sorts your clothes to align with your lifestyle activities.
- It maximises garments and enables you to form a defined personal style because, where possible, you can tweak outfits per level, not activity.
- Level 3 is your core style, which can be dressed up or down a level or two to appropriately align with any occasion in your life.
- Level dressing eliminates panic shopping or stress about what to wear in unexpected, unusual, rare or unplanned scenarios.

Suggested Actions

Thinking only about your Level 3 dress code, answer these three questions:

1. What are you dressing for during your daily routine? For example, F/T work, P/T work, Carer/Mum, leisure, etc.
2. Where do you spend most of your daily time? Office/site location, home, outside, other
3. Do you interact with other people? Yes, Sometimes, No.

Note your answers in the table. We will refer to your answers when making outfit combinations in Chapter 6.

What are you dressing for? Your levels of dress code will guide you.

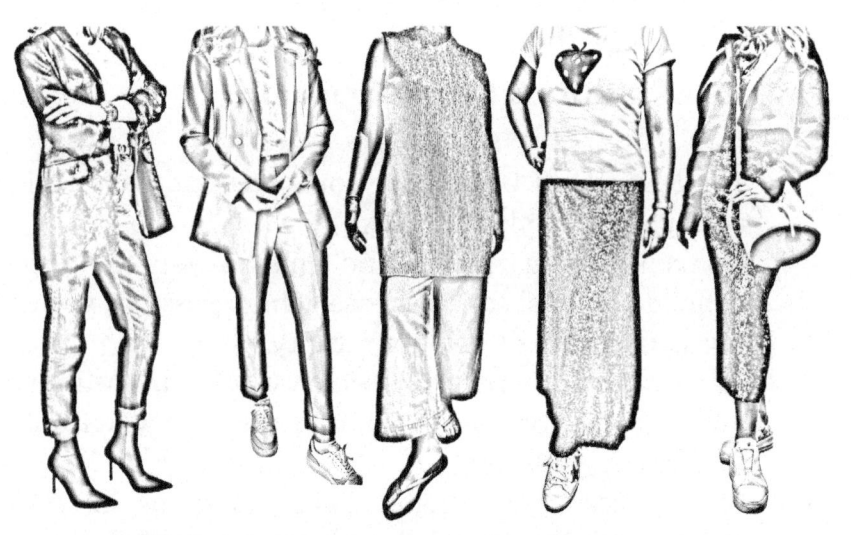

5'5" Size08 | 5'9" Size10 | 5'7" Size14 | 5'5" Size12 | 5'6" Size12

Level Dressing maximises garments across lifestyle – Sequins suitable for all levels

Your 5 Levels of Dress Code

5 — **Top Occasion**
I Wear Outfits for:
....
....
....

4 — **Dress Up**
I Wear Outfits for:
....
....
....

3 — **Base Level**
I Wear Outfits for:
....
....
....

2 — **Dress Down**
I Wear Outfits for:
....
....
....

1 — **Lounge Wear**
I Wear Outfits for:
....
....
....

4.2 Adapting Dress Codes

Once you know what you are dressing for, you have a functional clarity to hone in on, which helps define your personal style and teaches you how to maximise your style within your levels.

Getting your Level 3 nailed is vital in enabling you to adapt outfits up or down levels through finishing styling and using accessories. Levelling up and down can be as little as changing a pair of shoes, switching out a top, or replacing a hoodie with a jacket. The focus on caring about dressing well at Level 3 will give you the confidence to style for any occasion without the need to start from scratch. You will also avoid ending up with a make-do outfit that doesn't feel like you.

If your base Level 3 is not aligned with your lifestyle, it will skew the whole process and make it difficult to level up or down. This happened to Becky.

Becky works from home four days a week. Her flexible working hours mean she can taxi her kids around, regularly block out an hour in the day to exercise and pick up groceries on her travels. Her communication channels with work colleagues are generally screen shares. It didn't take long for Becky to form a daily habit of wearing her gym attire, even on the days she wasn't exercising, and throwing over a sweater for her work Zoom meetings. Becky had slipped into her Level 2 dress code - what I call the danger zone.

So what? You might be thinking. I'll tell you.

Becky had no differentiation between what she wore or how she felt about her work life, doing chores, leisure time, or fitness schedule. Even worse, when she was invited to attend a work meeting to be introduced to her new boss, Becky was unprepared to dress accordingly. On their first meeting, Becky entered the room and reached her hand forward to go in for the handshake with Angela, her new boss.

Immediately, Angela jerked back, withdrawing her hand, and sputtered, "Do your clothes belong to you?"

But it wasn't that Becky was wearing her gym kit, quite the opposite. Months of wearing stretchy waistbands and slouchy sweaters had not only created a sloppy dress code but had masked gradual weight gain. When Becky went to find something more appropriate from her wardrobe -

somewhere between Levels 3 and 4 - she wasn't expecting to find unflattering clothes that were too tight and looked snug. Panic buying struck. As if the pressure to find something new, buy a bigger size, and step out of her habitual comfort Level 2 dressing zone wasn't enough, what followed the awkward handshake at that first meeting was definitely not part of Becky's plan.

Unbeknownst to Becky, hanging from her jacket's inside arm seam was a shop security tag. Even worse, it had started leaking a red, inky substance that was about to splatter on whatever was in its path—the new Boss' pale mint green satin crepe blouse.

Thankfully, the red splatter landed safely on a few papers covering the desk, and after the initial embarrassment, the ladies found the funny side and now have a great working relationship.

Working with Becky on her dress codes means she now loves her Levels' ease. She keeps her gym wear firmly in Level 2, knows her Level 3 dress code is perfect for all her daily tasks, and often confidently dips into her Level 4 dress code when representing her company. Her level-up difference is often a third piece, such as a jacket or piece of jewellery or switching shoes.

Judi, who I introduced to you earlier, has a very subtle

difference between her levels. Rarely seen out of her jeans, the variation between Level 3 to Level 2 is only visible during seasonal changes when the temperature dictates sandals or boots, warm layers, or thinner tops. Level 4 is subtle, too—still jeans, but no frayed hems. Tops become more fitted, and she adds details such as a French tuck exposing a coloured belt with footwear choices that match the occasion. Judi's Level 5 is jaw-dropping. She loves a full-length dress of the strapless or sleeveless kind to which she adds multiple bracelets and bangles. Shoes remain the same as Level 4, and then she uses wraps and soft jackets from Levels 3 and even Level 2 to complete the look.

Formal, casual, and switching between the two, as well as being comfortable, stylish, and appropriately dressed for the occasion, is possible if you adopt this Level Code method.

<small>Example of lifestyle activities and what level of dress code is needed</small>

Example Lifestyle Activities

Recurring Life Situations - Monthly

Morning routine	30x	Level 1
Working from Home/Office	8x	Level 3
Working with Clients/Meetings	8x	Level 3
Presentations/Filming/Pitching	4x	Level 3/4
Evenings at home	20x	Level 2
Tasks around the house	8x	Level 2
Errands/Visiting	8x	Level 3
Exercise	12x	Level 2
Weekend/Outdoor activities	8x	Level 2/3
Casual social events	10x	Level 3/4
Occasional social events	1x	Level 5
Sleeping	30x	Level 1

5 Levels Of Dress Code - Summary

- The benefits of adapting your dress code between Levels means you do not need an entirely separate collection of clothes for different aspects of your life.
- You can invest in the stylish pieces you want because you know they will get worn, and your clothes

wardrobe will be easier to manage.
- People don't ask, "What shall I wear to walk the dog?". They ask, "What can I wear so I don't need to get fully changed after walking the dog?" Or how to dress to feel appropriately dressed to combine dog walking and a chore.
- The 5 Levels of Dress Code align your clothing and lifestyle, making it easier to develop a personal style.
- If implemented properly, the method eradicates the feeling of having nothing to wear and maintains your personal style, whatever you are dressing for.
- It also makes buying new clothes more successful. Just knowing you have something suitable to wear already gives you the best mindset and headspace to only buy something new if you see something better.
- Panic buying or choosing sub-par pieces can be eradicated.
- You'll have enough time to make sure that any embarrassing shop tags or labels have been removed!

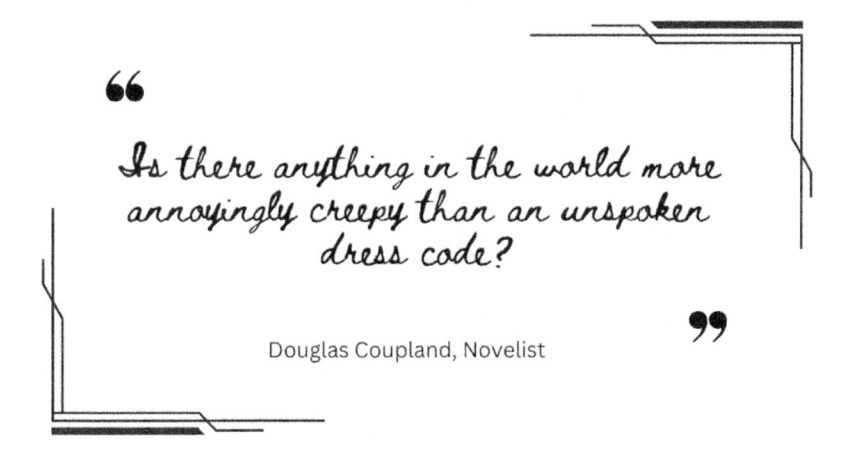

> *Is there anything in the world more annoyingly creepy than an unspoken dress code?*
>
> Douglas Coupland, Novelist

Suggested Actions

Make a list of your current lifestyle activities, alongside which Level of clothing you currently wear for each activity. Consider if that Level could go up one to make daily dressing easier. Think:

1. Are you dressing in an established style at Level 3, or have you slipped into Level 2?
2. Do you have items in Level 3 that you can style up to Level 4?
3. Do you have items in Level 2 that you can style up to Level 3?

Your Lifestyle Activities

Recurring Life Situations - Monthly

Activity	Frequency	
Morning routine	30x	Level
	x	Level
	x	Level
	x	Level
	x	Level
	x	Level
	x	Level
	x	Level
	x	Level
	x	Level
	x	Level
	x	Level

4.3 Your UPS Explained

Whatever you focus on will grow, including your Unique Personal Style, aka UPS.

We have talked about the fact that avoiding a full-length mirror, not paying attention, or wearing the same few items without any thought other than, "I've got clothes on," does not eliminate you from being seen or excuse you from exposing a visual language that will be seen and judged.

Your UPS is already out there, so why not focus on it as you dress daily to ensure it is a UPS that makes you feel good?

To delve deeper into the spectrum of what UPS means, here's a breakdown:

U = Unique

Being the only one of its kind, unlike anything else. Which is exactly what you are.

I'm going to kick off uniqueness by referencing celebrity fashion guru Trinny as an example.

Trinny can style out anything you put in front of her. A little tuck here, a ruche with a pin-brooch there, swish back that bit or even turn your shirt upside down and back-to-front (she does actually do that!). The whole performance, which usually starts by telling us she's been to her lock-up, is *so* watchable you can't wait to see what she does next.

The question is, "Would *you* wear it like Trinny?"

If you are a Trinny fan, you are likely to buy into her make-up range and settle for the entertainment of wondering what she will style next whilst implementing a few of her tips into your wardrobe if you have a piece that directly resonates.

Remember, though, you are just as unique as Trinny, and once you are in your wardrobe, you will find your own way to style outfits.

P = Personal

Belonging to or affecting a particular person rather than anyone else.

Style is undoubtedly personal and not all glamour, even at the world's most prestigious events. British costume designer Jenny Beavan, who won an Oscar in 2016, graciously collected her award wearing a regular black M&S jacket, black slacks and a red scarf. It was not the usual dress code for the Oscars, but it was Jenny's personal Level 5 dress code, as she told the world who were watching. Dressing up at glitzy galas is not her thing, she said. That didn't stop her style choice for making headline news, though, which shows that you can't 'opt' out of your personal style. Whatever you choose to wear conveys a message that tells a story.

By contrast, Emily Blunt sent the 2024 Oscar style critiques crazy when she dazzled in a sparkling beaded champagne-colour Schiaparelli gown which had floating shoulder straps – a deliberate fit feature that was intended not to fit but hover and a midsection embellishment in the shape of 'Y'-fronts. Yep, you read that correctly. Worth an internet search if you've not seen it. More proof that style is a matter of personal taste whilst still being a visual language that sets tongues wagging.

The point here is that *you* can control what the wagging tongues say about you.

S = Style

> *A distinctive appearance and how you express yourself to the world.*

Your Style of clothing tells your story. Have you noticed how the most successful newsreaders wear plain colours? As do politicians and royals.

Monochromatic dressing can keep an audience engaged regardless of whether they are bright colours, bold colours, modern or concise colours. Adding patterns mixes colours, which can make the boldness (of the monochrome dressing) lose its concise feel. Perhaps it's worth keeping patterns for off-duty clothing and the more plain for work? As I've mentioned, that's what we see most often with the Royals and politicians.

There's nothing wrong with using bold colours and/or patterns; it's just a case of tweaking these as required for audience and level. If you need your audience to concentrate and maintain focus, bold patterns are best avoided.

The message here about Style is that you use your style - how you express yourself to the world - as another part of your story. Like those Oscars outfits, your Style affects how the world sees and reacts to you.

UPS – Summary

- Your UPS is a measure of consistency to detail and an acceptance that what you wear is an expression of you and how you are seen by others.
- If you ignore detail and fail to be consistent, the result will be ill-fitting, sloppy, non-committal dressing - and

that is how the world will view you.

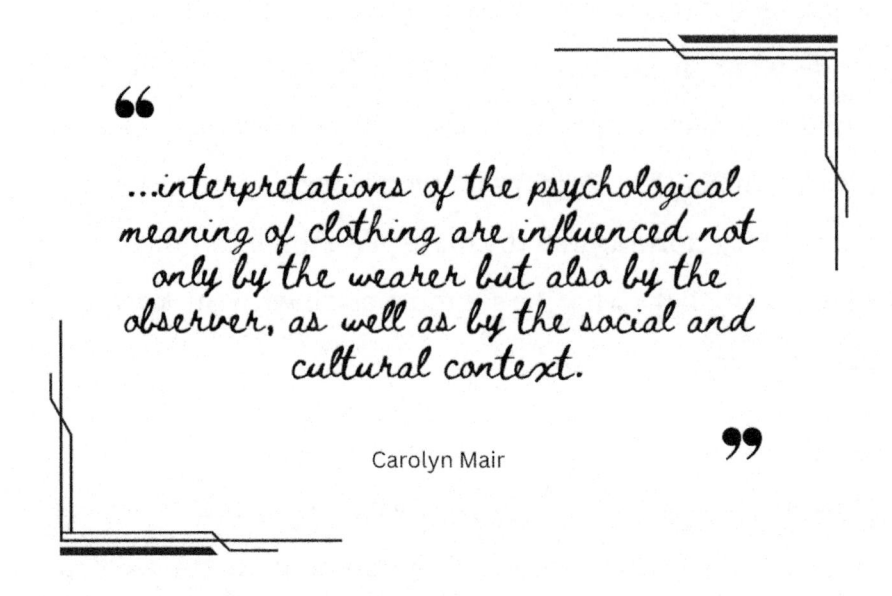

> ...interpretations of the psychological meaning of clothing are influenced not only by the wearer but also by the observer, as well as by the social and cultural context.
>
> Carolyn Mair

Suggested Actions

We are about to enter your wardrobe and transform it into the best collection of clothes it can possibly be. We won't stop there, either. This process starts an ongoing cycle that will become a joyous, integral part of your life.

The only action required here is to ask:

"Are you ready to manage your clothes and be stylish forever?"

175

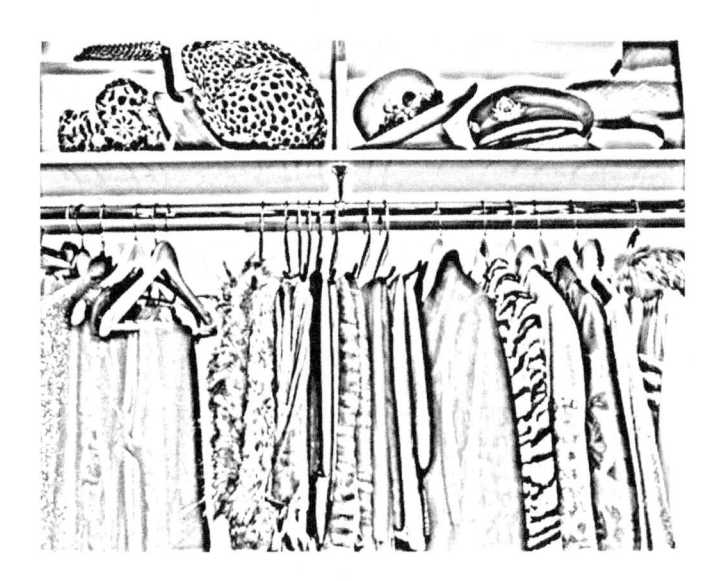

5. Wardrobe Therapy

- Part 1

Sort Your Clothes Out

Wardrobe Therapy starts by looking at what you already have and sorting these out. You are looking to unearth your best bits which will be what we use for your true starting point. Once you have sorted these pieces from the rest of your collection, you will find it so much easier to evolve your style and move it forwards in an informed direction.

The first step of Wardrobe Therapy is to undertake a Wardrobe Audit, which is exactly the same process for all sizes of clothing and collections. The only difference is the duration of the process which will differ depending upon how many clothes are in your collection.

Things We Are Going To Consider As We Start Your Wardrobe Audit:

1. Too much of anything rarely makes you feel good - the same applies to your clothes. I've worked with wardrobes that simply contain far too many clothes, so everything becomes a blur. At first sight, it can appear impossible to tease out what constitutes a 'best item', let alone find any common thread to define even the hint of a style. If this is your wardrobe, don't worry. I've got you!
2. At the opposite end of the clothes collection spectrum is the minimalist wardrobe. This limited collection relies on pieces mixing and matching with each other and usually involves a repeat buying habit.
3. Then there is everything in between.

Neither type of wardrobe is right or wrong; there isn't an

optimum number of clothes we should own. However, there is a system that fits all wardrobes, which is what we are going to learn now.

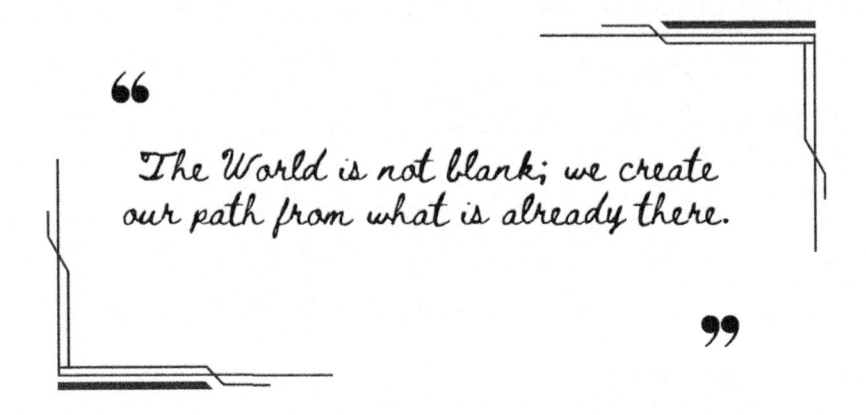

> *The World is not blank; we create our path from what is already there.*

One final thought before we begin. If you've ever said, *"I wish I'd kept that,"* about an item you have moved on from – it's immaterial. If you *had* kept it, you still wouldn't be wearing it now because what you are remembering is how it used to make you feel and look. That feeling is also from the past, and it is unlikely it would be recreated if that item were in your possession now. Like everything, we only remember the good, so it's easy to pretend that an item was and would be perfect simply because we have no way to prove it now.

And so, without further ado (grand fanfare!), it's time to
OPEN YOUR WARDROBE and
SORT OUT YOUR CLOTHES!

5.1 Wardrobe Therapy – How to Audit Your Wardrobe

---•---

A Wardrobe Audit is the preliminary decluttering stage, during which you filter out everything that doesn't fit you, is damaged, is unwearable in its current state, or you simply don't love anymore. It is also a stock-take to remind you what you have.

Every wardrobe is different and the suggested timings I have included here are based on my experience working with clients. Most people find it a very therapeutic experience, and I'm sure you will too. Hence, I like to call the entire process, Wardrobe Therapy.

You will need:

You Will Need:

1. Clothes Rail
2. Tote Bag - for clothes needing repair or alteration
3. Large Bag - for charity donations
4. Large clear plastic storage box – for items to sell
5. Notebook and Pen
6. 2-4 hours of time

1. To begin, take each item out of your wardrobe, one by one, and ask these 3 questions, answering only YES or NO

YES or NO

1. Does the garment fit you today? *(Not sure, refer to Chapter 2, Fabric v Cut)*
2. Do you love it 100% and it makes you feel good when you put it on?
3. Is the garment in excellent condition without the need for repair or alteration?

This 'YES/NO' process should be actioned quickly and is for every individual garment.

If you answer **YES to all three questions**, with no 'buts' or hesitations, place the item on a hanger on the rail.

If you answer **YES to the first two questions but NO to question three**, place the item in the 'repairs' tote bag. Use your notebook and pen to list the repair items and what repair or alteration is needed.

If you answer **NO to questions (a) or (b), you have two options**:

> Either place the item in the charity donation bag
> or add it to your 'to sell' box.

Reselling clothes on the pre-loved market is entirely your choice and is usually determined by the time invested to do it and the money made. As a brief guide:

> ~ Low-end items like Primark, New Look, and supermarket brands will only fetch £1-£2 resale.
> ~ H&M and Zara are approximately £3-£15.
> ~ Higher-end brands such as Reiss, and Mint Velvet will likely sell for £15 plus.
> ~ Designers like Scamp & Dude, ME+EM will usually sell for more.

At this stage (and for time efficiency), if it's not a higher-end item, pop it in the donations bag. You don't need to give away today or part with anything you don't want to.

2. If you have items in drawers or a second wardrobe, keep going until you've gone through all your clothes or when 3 hours are up.

If you haven't completed all your clothes within 3 hours, then stop and book another session into your diary, preferably within the same week.
I have worked with many women with large wardrobes, and after 3 hours, the quick-fire process is no longer effective because the volume of clothes building up on the rail and the donation/sell bags become distracting.
So, stop and make sure you book a continuation session in your diary.

3. When you have completed or reached the 3-hour mark, use the next hour to tidy your space, starting with your main wardrobe.

Your wardrobe, or at least a large proportion of it, should now be empty, and any non-wardrobe items need to be taken out and stored elsewhere in their appropriate places.

4. Use this opportunity to give your wardrobe a good clean.

Dust it out and pop the hoover round.

5. Place the items from the rail that have all passed the three questions with a **YES** back into your cleansed wardrobe, neatly on hangers, or neatly folded if going

on a shelf or in a drawer.

6. Next, address your alterations notebook. Did you discover any items you've replaced in your wardrobe that you will use instead of those you've put out for repair/alteration? If yes, it's not worth going ahead with the alteration, so remove those items from the bag.

Are there any other items you don't love enough to spend money and effort on getting them repaired or altered? If yes, remove those too.

The remaining items, along with the notes of repair/alteration, need to be dropped off with your local seamstress as soon as possible. (Refer back to Chapter 2.3 if it's your first time using a seamstress).

7. Now, go through your donations pile and double-check that you are happy to move the items on. Decide which of these you want to donate and which you would like to sell.

If you are hesitant about an item, put it at the bottom of the donation pile to give yourself some extra thinking time.

DO NOT put anything from this pile back in your wardrobe – it is not a 10/10 perfect piece because it did not pass the three-question test.

Decide which charity shop you are going to donate your surplus items to and give yourself a date and time when you will drop them off or arrange for them to be collected.

8. Go through the items you have selected to sell and check whether they are really sellable. Consider the time you will need to invest in the selling process and compare this with your potential income.

If you are new to selling pre-loved and/or unsure if this is for you, then simply switch these pieces to the donation bag.

There are alternatives to online selling, such as pre-loved clothing agencies, which I will discuss in more detail later. For now, the main thing is to decide what you are going to do with your surplus items and make a plan. If you don't have a plan, you will be tempted to put some of these items back into your wardrobe, so ensure you put a date in your diary for disposing of these surplus items however you choose to do this.

Do not keep anything for just-in-case purposes. This doesn't happen; these clothes will just clutter up your space and confuse your style.

Outerwear, Underwear & Functional Clothing
The same process can be used for your coats, footwear, gym wear, underwear, and any other category of clothes in your life. Remove every item one piece at a time, answer the three questions above, clean your space, put back what you are keeping, and bag up everything else.

You will notice there will be an additional 'throw-away' pile, too. Shoes, gym wear, functional wear, and underwear are often worn until they wear out, so they are likely to make up the bulk of this pile. You will also add those items you have decided not to repair to this pile, too. Throwing clothes out as waste is the last resort. Some places recycle the fibres of worn-out textiles, including leather and plastic, and there are countless clothes recycling centres you can also use.

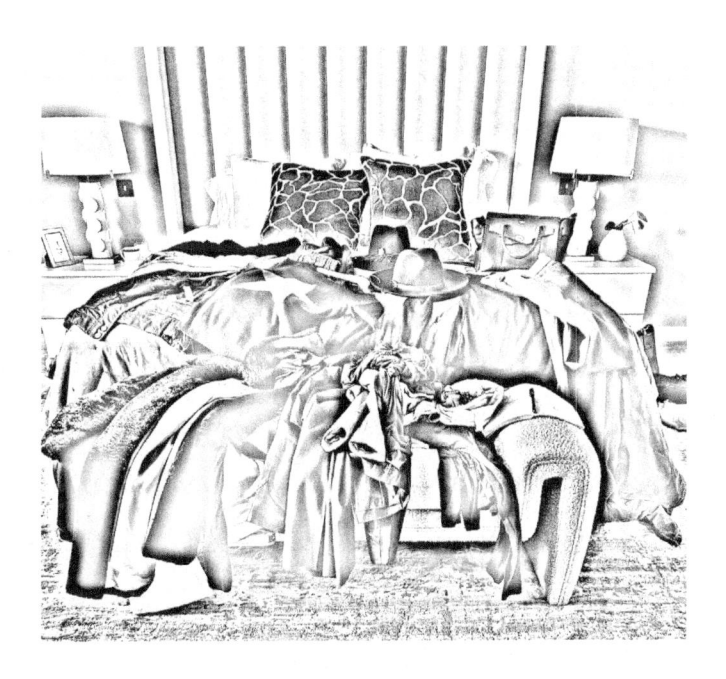

Unaccounted Items

Ah, yes. Despite your best efforts, there will be some items that:

- Don't fit you today, but it will at some point.
- They are sentimental pieces.

- You love and can't move on, but know you are unlikely to wear.

It is your choice to have these items in your life; just don't have them in your wardrobe. Ironically, these pieces of sentiment or fond memory-provoking garments detract value from your day-to-day dressing. They are often why you get stuck with what to wear even though you have a full wardrobe.

One of my clients, Fern, had accumulated a host of sentimental wardrobe items after her mum passed away. The collection contained prized pieces which had belonged to her grannie, too and knowing that Fern's mum had carefully kept these pieces and occasionally worn them herself, Fern could not move them on. Instead, given that these items were vintage and came from a bygone era, Fern contacted Esther, a costume maker with contacts who worked on Netflix and BBC dramas. Fern's family heirlooms are now part of the period costumes department and have been featured in Sister Boniface on the BBC. The fur hat used - also known as "Joy" - was named after Fern's granny.

Theatres, TV, film, and amateur dramatic groups are always looking for authentic fabrics, trims, clothing, and accessories, so if you have any of these, start asking around. You'll be able to find a local contact who can advise you on how your sentimental heirlooms might be able to live on.

Wardrobe Audit – Summary

- The benefit of a full clothes audit before any styling takes place is to declutter and filter out what doesn't add value to your daily dressing.
- Set aside sessions of 4-hour blocks, using 3 hours to audit and 1 hour to tidy your space, and then plan what you will do with the surplus.
- Go through your entire clothes collection, which includes coats, footwear, accessories, and anything else.
- Remember, you are just answering the three questions at this first Auditing stage of Wardrobe Therapy.

Suggested Actions

If you want to manage your clothes, dress confidently, and nail your style, don't wait. Reach for your diary, source a rail, and get some bags ready right now.

TOP-TIPS:
If this is something you have done before but are finding it difficult to know what to keep and what to move on, try doing it with a friend.
I say this because from my experience working with clients who have decluttered before instructing my services, we have had to do a further declutter, and here's why:

Your clothes are your closest possessions, and they carry memories your subconscious cannot forget. This includes

how well certain garments have served you in the past, making you believe they might serve you well again in the future. If you have a friend present, they can point this out.

Other Factors That Cloud Judgement:

Designer Brands
Hanging on to a piece just because it's a designer brand or a high price tag is not of value if it doesn't fit you or is not your style. You can sell it and put the funds towards your perfect pieces. (Refer to Chapter 2.4 Worth, Value & Cost if you need a Reminder).

Gifts
Saving someone else's feelings by holding on to an item just because they gave it to you, will not help you with your style. You're not wearing it anyway so how do they know if it's still in your wardrobe or not? Move it on and let someone else enjoy wearing it.

Fit
Be honest with the fit. Just because you can get the zip done up doesn't mean it fits you properly or comfortably. (Chapter 2.1 – Fabric & Cut, is all about how fabric and cut affect a garment's fit).

Items to Move On

Repeat Items	If original is worn out only keep the replacement. If a uniform or functional underlayer store together and regularly check condition. Any other reason, just keep the best one.
Just-in-case Items	These pieces add unnecessary clutter. Refer to your lifestyle activities and if items are not required today, move them out and donate to charity.
Sentimental Items	If they are not relevant to your daily dressing, store somewhere else, not in your daily wardrobe space.
Expensive Labels & Brands	If they don't meet your criteria of YES to the 3 questions, they are not right for you. Sell, and put the money towards a perfect item.
Gifts	Are you keeping it to avoid upsetting the person who gifted it? They would prefer you to sell it and choose something you love and will wear.
Wedding Dresses & One-offs	You will not wear it again. Store it elsewhere, or have it made into something else, or sell it while it is still fresh.
Items that are too small	You can't wear them today; therefore, they are cluttering up your wardrobe space with no purpose. If they will fit in the future, store them elsewhere for a set amount of time.
Items that are too big	They don't fit; therefore, they cannot be worn. Have them altered if you love them or sell them.
Damaged Items	You can't wear them in their current condition. Get the repair job done or donate to clothes recycling.
Items needing alteration	You can't wear them in their current form. Get the alteration completed or move the garment on as is.

5.2 Clothes Storage Space

Whatever your space is, don't be afraid to change it around. Just because you allocated drawers or wardrobe space to certain items ten years ago doesn't mean it still works. The aim is to make all your clothes easily accessible with what you dress for most - Level 3, at your fingertips.

Here's A Guide To Sorting Out Your Clothing Space And Storage:

1. Start by assessing every space you have available for your clothes. Don't forget coats, shoes, and bags. Acknowledge how much hanging, shelf, and drawer space you have and work out whether it is all together in one room or if there are various rooms you can use for storage.

2. Do you share a wardrobe with a partner? Check if their allocated space is being used efficiently, or can you swap it around with yours?

3. Are your coats and footwear kept somewhere else? If yes, are they mixed in with the rest of your family's coats and footwear and a few non-clothing items, too?

4. The ideal is to have all your clothes in one place, or at least all *your* things grouped together if a space is shared. Some of my clients let their partners take the wardrobe in the bedroom and use another area better suited to the (amount of) items they have.

5. Apart from physical storage space, your wardrobe needs to be accessible and care for your items. For example, if you are folding items, expect them to crease; if you roll items, can you remember what they are? Can you see what's at the bottom of the pile if you stack folded items? Hanging space is best for everything except jumpers or stretchy/heavy fabrics that cause misshaping of the shoulders when hung on a hanger.

6. Items made from stretch or heavy fabrics can be switched to a clip hanger or a wide-cushioned hanger to prevent the misshaping.

7. Wide cushioned or wooden hangers take up a lot more space, so folding and storing them in a drawer or shelf compartment may be better for your space.

8. Regular cleaning of space is as important as keeping your clothes and items washed and dust-free.

Did you know that cleanliness is the number one preventer of moths? Clothes moths are attracted to dust and clothes stained with sweat and food. Once in your wardrobe, moths will munch away on your wool, cotton, linen, cashmere, alpaca, mohair, and silk items. In fact, almost any natural fibre – feathers, felt, leather - will do for a hungry little moth larva. It's not just your jumpers that need to be protected; your shoes and accessories need a dust down and polish, too.

9. If you are a cashmere or wool jumper wearer, seal your clean, folded knits in plastic zip-lock garment bags – these can be purchased from places like Argos or Amazon. You can also buy anti-moth paper liners or cedarwood balls, both of these slip nicely into your drawers and add protection.

A regular swish around your wardrobe with the vacuum cleaner is often enough to disturb the build-up of dust and the little moth blighters as well!

10. To maximise hanging space use thin, non-slip, hangers. Prioritise your go-to Level 3 items in the middle of your wardrobe, even if they are t-shirts that you are used to storing in a drawer. Put your Level 4 and 5 items at each end of your wardrobe – like bookends. Level 1 clothes and most of Level 2 (depending on your lifestyle) will be the folded or rolled items, which ensures that everything is accessible without causing a clothes avalanche when you're pulling out what to wear.

11. After your Audit, you may have empty areas. Check if more hanging space or folding space is needed and whether it is possible to adapt your wardrobe.

12. If space is limited and you simply have more clothes than you can store, it is time to consider the Pareto principle, aka the 20/80 rule. We wear 20% of our clothes 80% of the time. Can you scale back any further? I've said and implied all the way through this book that the more you can limit and drill down to

what clothes look, feel, and work best for you, the easier dressing becomes and the more confident you will be in evolving your style.

13. Some clients use vacuum-packed bags to store out-of-season clothes. Although this can be a space-saving option, it adds another layer to clothes management and can interrupt the flow of Level dressing. Consider if you've just accumulated too many clothes in this case. Can you re-audit your collection to check?

14. Do not mistake a tidy space for an organised one. I have been called upon many a time to help women who have immaculate-looking wardrobes with every item they own beautifully hung, folded, and compartmentalised, yet they still need help putting outfits together and remaining stylish with fresh looks.

Guide To Storage (Based On Level)

Adjust depending on your lifestyle and in accordance with your clothing types:

Level 3 - Hang in the middle, the most accessible part of your go-to wardrobe.

Levels 4 and 5 - Are the 'bookends' of your hanging space, placed at each of the rail. This is because they are not accessed as much as your Level 3 items.

Levels 1 and 2 – Can be hung if space is available or folded and placed in drawers, shelves etc.

Items not to be hung - knits, jumpers, sweaters and any stretchy or heavy fabrics that become misshapen by hangers.

Clothes And Storage Space - Summary

- Assess your space and portion it according to the amount and type of clothes you have.
- Don't be afraid to move clothes around or store them differently to suit what you have now, rather than continuing to place items by habit.
- Hang your clothes using (where possible) thin, non-slip hangers and larger, stronger or wooden hangers for coats.
- Delicate or heavy fabrics may need to be hung on padded hangers to avoid misshapen shoulders or upside down on clip hangers. If folding, rolling, or stacking clothes, ensure you can still see and access them easily.
- Regularly hoover your clothes storage spaces to eliminate dust and disturb clothes moths. Cedarwood balls or hangers and anti-moth drawer liners are recommended if you have natural fibre fabrics.

Suggested Actions

After your audit, allocate storage space for what you have and reallocate areas (if needed) when space is freed up post-audit.

195

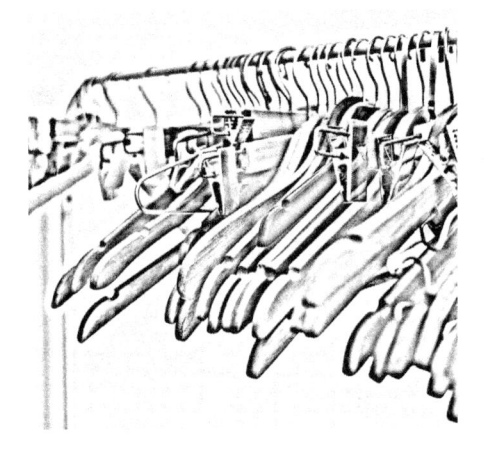

5.3 Nothing to Wear, Feeling Thread Bare

In this section, I want to reassure you that if your **NO** pile is *twice the volume of what you put back in your Wardrobe,* you will undoubtedly feel threadbare – which is perfectly normal.

Angie was 50 when I met her. Recently divorced after 23 years of marriage, the latter two years in a situation of separation while still sharing the family home along with their two sons, one of whom is severely disabled. Angie is great company to be around, yet by her own admission, she does not have much of a social life; every minute of her waking hours is taken with her work or children. She simply did not have the capacity or inclination to address her wardrobe. The problem was that her wardrobe contained size 10 clothes, and she was currently a size 14. Her most recent buys were a cream long-length jumper and black leggings purchased from supermarkets while doing her grocery shopping.

I met Angie by chance on a training course, and a Wardrobe Editor was the last person she thought she'd have anything in common with, but our friendship grew, and to her surprise and my delight, she eventually agreed to let me into her wardrobe. I won't sugar-coat it - the audit was tough. Rich brocade skirts, pin-tucked detailed blouses, embroidered chiffon gipsy tops, asymmetric necklines, textured fabrics, structured silhouettes… the most beautiful clothes, but all of them too small.

Then, the clothes that did fit her fell into two distinct categories: 1) the ones she wore - leggings, a long pale denim skirt, and a couple of long, shapeless cream jumpers. 2) and the ones in her new size 14 with the labels still attached.

It is fair to say it was the sparsest audit I had ever done. We went from a healthy-sized wardrobe full to the brim to just a few sets of below-mediocre clothes. But that wasn't the surprise. Angie knew full well she was wearing less than 5% of what she owned; the problem was she had been on 'getting-dressed pause' for so long that every aspect of what she loved about clothes, fabric, colour, shape silhouette had become out of her reach.

The same clothes in a bigger size were not an option, or she would have already done that. Together, we established Angie's daily dressing needs, what she was dressing for, including her Level 3 lifestyle, clothing styles she had loved in the past and why, and what she wished she could wear now, and we devised a plan.

She loved strong colours, structured fabrics, and detailed finishes - the very opposite of the cream jumper and leggings - but more in keeping with her previous beautiful wardrobe. The solution was simply silhouettes in the fabrics she loved.

To get Angie on board with looking at her new body shape and find outfit silhouettes that made her feel good, we started with underwear. Angie had revealed she had no idea how to cope with new wobbly bits that her younger self didn't have – I introduced her to SPANX®, support tights and booked her into a bra fitting. We moved away from trousers and tops to avoid the issue of top lengths and focused on dresses. We selected darker, richer-coloured fabrics with simple patterns or unusual necklines. Now, Angie had some confidence that she could choose and wear beautiful clothes again, and she revealed her magnificent handbag collection! We chose footwear and soft jackets that worked with dresses and long skirts, pairing each outfit with a handbag for detail and creating her signature look.

Holding on to clothes that no longer fit your body or lifestyle skews where you are now with your wardrobe. Unfortunately, opting for *'I won't bother with style until I have time'* simply isn't an option. It pushes you further away from where you want to be and conveys a visual language that isn't your story.

I introduced Angie to Vinted, where she gladly sells her cherished, pre-loved size 10s to new owners who she hopes will get the same joy from them as she did. She uses her earnings to focus on her new shopping list of stylish clothes.

Every wardrobe is different and depending on how many clothes you own and how honest you are with filtering out what no longer serves you, you might feel a little threadbare - but you weren't wearing those clothes anyway. If you truly want to own a stylish wardrobe that is easy to manage, makes you feel good, and is mood-lifting, this process will make it possible. Whether your Audit result is your best 50%, 20%, or 5%, by default, this will be your best 100% and is your ultimate starting point to progress and improve your style.

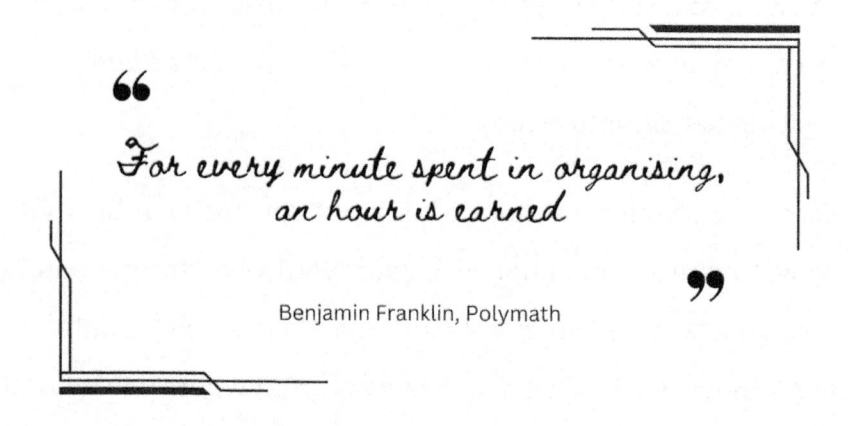

> *For every minute spent in organising, an hour is earned*
>
> Benjamin Franklin, Polymath

Before we move on to the next step, *'Editing and Adding to your Best'*, here's what to do with your unwanted items.

5.4 What to do with Surplus Clothes

All clothes and wardrobe items are recyclable. No clothing item needs to end up in a landfill.

The three options are:
1. Recycle
2. Donate
3. Sell.

All have varying time constraints, arrangements and availability depending on where you live.

Recycling

Locate your nearest recycling centre or clothes bank by searching online using the words textiles and shoes.

Re-purposing can be done too. T-shirt fabric and tights can be cut into cleaning rags for bicycles and outdoor patio furniture, for example.

Look out for annual projects, awareness days, and charity fundraisers. *Genetic Disorder UK* initiated 'Jeans for Genes' week, which inspires and supports local communities, colleges, and schools to put on fundraising events using unwanted denim donations. These events can range from using denim to make sculptures or organising re-fashioned clothing competitions. The aim is to raise money and awareness in a sustainable way.

Donations

Donating to Charity shops is quick and easy. To view the options in your area, use Google Maps and search for charity shops, thrift shops, or op shops.

If you have an M&S store nearby, you can donate to their *Shwopping Initiative* which is a joint venture with Oxfam to give unwanted clothes a new life.

If you have an H&M store, they will take a bag of unwanted clothes in return for a £5 gift voucher – something they have been offering since 2013.

If it sounds like an effort to drop your clothes off at these places (and others) you can book a collection. The list of companies that will collect is growing. A few of note are:

icollectclothes.co.uk
donateclothes.uk
recycle-more.co.uk
werecycleclothes.org.

There are even clothes-for-cash websites and apps like Anglo Doorstep. A Google search for 'collect unwanted clothes' will bring up the latest and nearest information about where you are.

Alternatively, you could organise your own *'Swish'*, a clothes-swapping event between friends or your community. I did my first one at my home and it completely took over the house for about a week as people dropped off bags of garments in advance. I had to clear the entire ground floor, hire rails, borrow hangers, and call upon a local cake baker to provide refreshments and help me out. I've since discovered local cafes and community spaces are always happy to host such events!

If that still sounds like too much effort, Olio is a free sharing app for local communities. It's designed to make it easy to give away the things you don't need to someone else who would value them.

General clothes are sought after everywhere, and there are many options to make it as easy as possible to donate your surplus items. However, do check what each charity accepts. Not all accept items such as shoes or bras, for example. If you have some items not accepted by your chosen charity, do an individual Google search. I recently did a search for 'unwanted pre-loved bras' and was presented with eleven options for donating or recycling these within seconds. The same happened with shoes. Whatever surplus you have to donate, Google search your area with your specific items.

Selling

The options for making money from unwanted clothes are vast, too; however, the buyer always gets a better deal than the seller, which is something to keep in mind.

Even if your item has never been worn, is in mint condition and has its original tags and packaging, it is still classed as a pre-loved item.

Let's have a quick look at a few of the sites accepting sales of pre-loved clothes (from low to high):

- Websites such as *Re-fashion* are technically donation sites, but like H&M, they will give you vouchers to spend in return for a bag full of donated items. There are restrictions on what they take; fast and ultra-fast fashion are not accepted.

- *Vinted* and *Depop* are both user-friendly mobile apps where clothes are sold for as little as £1. In my experience, the most popular selling price bracket is £5 - £40 because buyers are looking for bargains. With these types of apps, you need to give thought to how much time it will take you to photograph your items, upload them, package them and drop them off at collection points versus your potential income. If you do get into the pre-loved market this way, it does become addictive. I have many clients who love to sell cheap and buy cheap using these types of sites.

- *Facebook Marketplace*, another option, allows buyers to collect from your doorstep, eliminating the P&P time and expense. Don't assume this is quicker, though. Making arrangements for mutual collection times or buyers asking if you can deliver often happens, and vigilance is required because you are giving out your address and other details. Again, buyers are looking for a bargain and even a freebie giveaway, but it can be a great resource for unwanted items to be taken off your hands.

- *eBay* is an auction site, originally called AuctionWeb, when it was established in 1995. Here, a sought-after item can make you some unexpected money. A good way to check potential is to search for an item similar to what you are selling and then see how many 'bidders' and 'watchers' it has. If you are unfamiliar with how the auction works or unsure if your unwanted items will sell, this might not be the best option for you.

- *Vestiare Collective* is a favourite of mine for luxury brands and designer labels. One of the original contenders, it was founded in 2009, way before the surge of pre-loved fashion was a thing. I used to bag a

bargain from an eBay auction just to sell it at a profit on Vestiare. I even bought brand new designer goods in the sales at a 70% discount, confidently knowing I could make a profit on it! Those days are long gone, especially since superstars like Rhianna put pre-loved on the map.
- Pre-loved clothing Agencies and Boutiques are physical shops that take your unwanted clothes and re-sell them for a cut of the profit. On average, they take 50%-70%, which might sound like a lot, but the fact you don't have to invest any time other than dropping off your stuff and going back to collect your money makes this option, in my opinion, 100% worth it. This is another Google search to locate if you have a pre-loved agency in your area. In Cheltenham, there is an agency called Re-vamp. Glancing at the window, you'd never know it was pre-loved items; more about this gem and others like it later when we start sourcing your style. The point here is that the quality of the garments needs to be re-sellable at a certain price point to make them profitable for all.

The bottom line is that pre-loved is massive, and it is here to stay. If you have high-end brands, designer labels or genuine vintage items, it is worth investing your time to learn how to sell pre-loved or use a pre-loved dress agency. It's an entire subject of its own.

There are links on my website to ask about courses if you'd like to dig a little deeper into this subject: www.myvos.co.uk

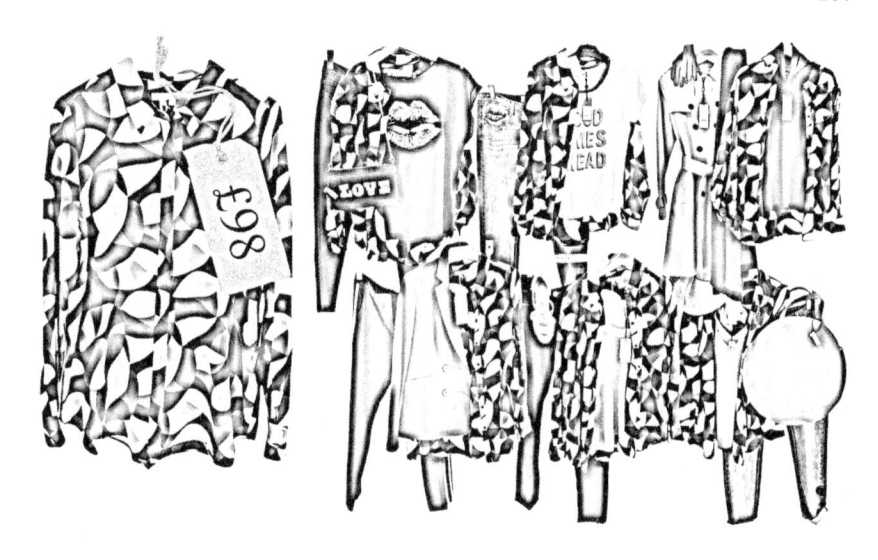

Silk Boden shirt, £98 new in 2019, sold for £55 in 2024

A silk shirt from a reputable brand that can be styled in multiple ways across levels, will hold its value.

Clothing Surplus - Summary

- Your surplus garments are in great demand. The pre-loved market is growing exponentially, as are charitable causes and fibre recycling options. All three areas rely on us being willing to move on our surplus, unwanted garments and in return we can help, support, and earn money whilst decluttering our wardrobes and ultimately improving our style.
- Be realistic, though. Selling is not an instant money maker. It takes effort to familiarise yourself with the functionality of the sites and learn the tricks to maximise price, all without a guarantee that the time spent was worth the money earned.
- Donating clothes is much easier, and with lots of charities collecting directly from your doorstep, moving clothes ethically is accessible to all.

Suggested Actions

Prepare what you will do with your surplus items to prevent them from sneaking back into your wardrobe space.

1. Compare pre-loved sites to see if you like the interface and ease of navigation. Use the search filters like a regular website for dress size, brand label, colour, and style.
2. If you like it, set up your profile to sell and buy.
3. Search for pre-loved dress agencies, charity shops, thrift stores and op shops so that you know what's available in your area and restrictions on what they will take.
4. Locate your local clothes bank.

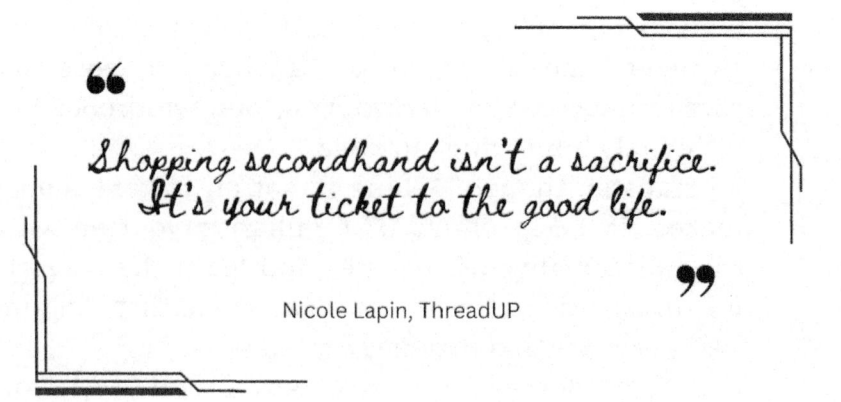

> Shopping secondhand isn't a sacrifice. It's your ticket to the good life.
>
> Nicole Lapin, ThreadUP

6. Wardrobe Therapy

- Part 2

Clothes Into Outfits

You can't wear a top without a bottom, and even a one-and-done jumpsuit needs shoes. Remember how we talked in Chapter 2 about how one garment does not make a wearable outfit? Now that we have sorted out our clothes, the next step is to make all of those audited pieces into outfits. In this chapter, we will look at how to turn your garments into a multitude of ready-to-wear outfits and maximise each piece.

Once an outfit is put together, you can swap out one item or add a piece to make an entirely new outfit, and by following this method, you will be able to identify missing items or more pieces, which, when added to your collection, will create further outfits in your style. Swapping pieces into and out of an outfit enables you to move up and down between your Levels of Dress Code, too, which justifies investment buys and, above all, maintains your true style.

It's time now to practice your own Levels of Dress Code. To do this, we will need to refer back to the notes you made in previous chapters. The key is to recall what is important to you so that you can ensure that the outfits we are now going to create, really do reflect your style.

Let's edit your audited clothes!

> *No matter how you feel, get up, dress up and show up*
>
> Regina Brett, Inspirational Speaker

6.1 Wardrobe Therapy – How to Edit Your Clothes

You will need 2 hours of uninterrupted time and a pale tablecloth or sheet.

1. Pull out your five favourite items from your audited wardrobe. Those of you who have really been paying attention will remember that I asked you to look at five pieces in Chapter 2 when we were talking about fabrics. If the five pieces you chose in Chapter 2 have made it through to this stage of your audit, then add these pieces to the five favourites you select now.

2. Select one top and create an outfit that you could wear now or tomorrow. To make your first outfit, you can include any of your audited clothes from your wardrobe or any of your other five selected favourite items.

3. Add footwear and any layers that are needed to make

the outfit suitable for the season both inside and outside.

4. You are creating an outfit for your base Level 3, which should be appropriate for how you spend most of your time.

Be honest here with your day-to-day lifestyle needs. A casual look still needs to be polished and thought through. Even if you spend most of your time at home or aren't in the company of other people, you still need to formulate an outfit that is your visual language. (If you wear a uniform for work, this will be slightly different, so base your Levels of Dress Code on your off-duty activities).

5. Check your completed finished outfit and make sure that it:

Creates an overall silhouette that balances your body shape – revisit Chapter 1.4, Body Beautiful, if you need a recap.

Consists of shapes proportionate in length and width for your height – revisit Chapter 1.5, Switching Focus from Body to Clothes

Is constructed from fabrics which enhance your figure – if you need a fabric reminder, Chapter 2.1, Fabric & Cut explains.

Has a neckline shape and garment details you love – see notes you made in Chapter 1.2, Style History, and Chapter 3.3, Style Personality.

Includes footwear and top layers which are of the same level as the Dress Code – refer to your tables in Chapter 4, Daily Dress Code.

6. Lay your outfit out flat on the pale cloth. This is referred to as a 'Flat Lay' or 'Flat Styling' and is a quick method of formulating outfit ideas rather than taking up valuable

time getting changed and trying items on.

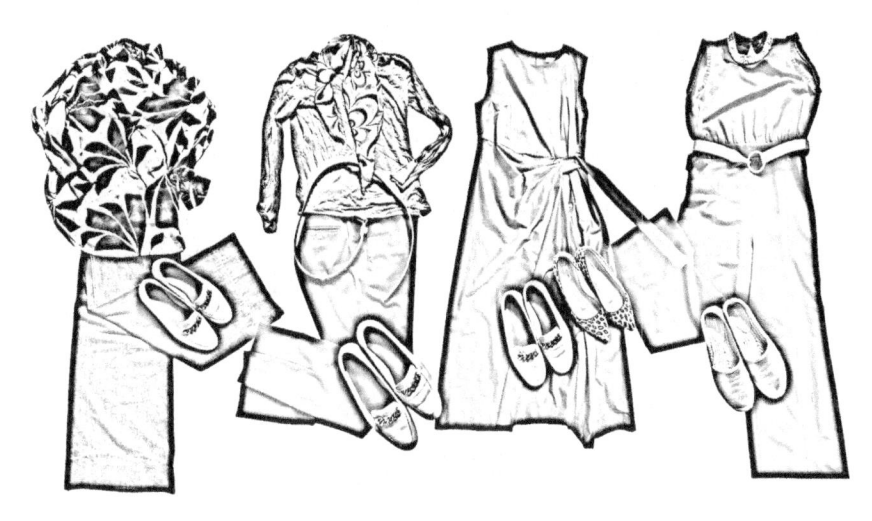

Flat-lay styling is a quick method of formulating lots of ready-to-wear outfit ideas. Image Chapter 6.1

7. Take two photos of your flat lay. The first one should show how you would wear this outfit inside, and the second photo should show it styled with the outer layer/coat as you would wear it outside.

216 | 2ND SKIN

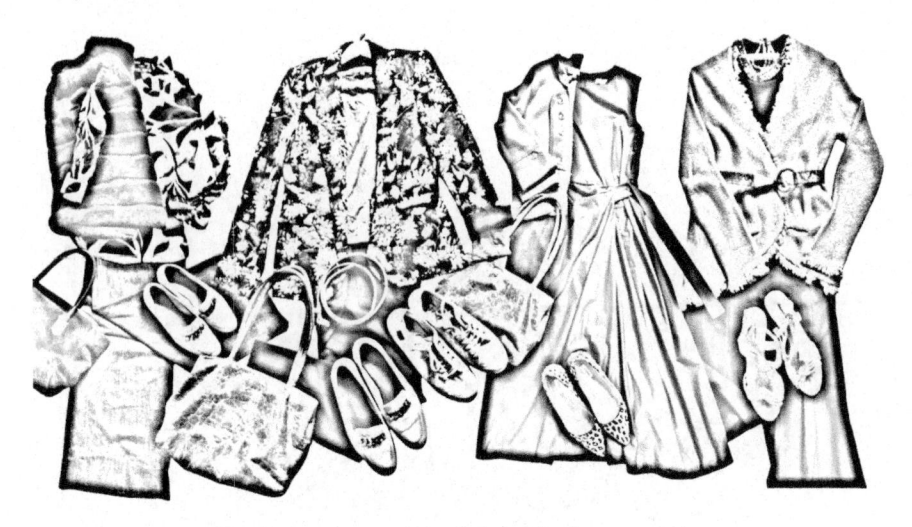

Add outerwear, accessories and alternative footwear options.

SCAN TO VIEW REAL WOMEN
OUTFIT LIBRARY

8. Next, switch out one item at a time and make as many outfits as you like.

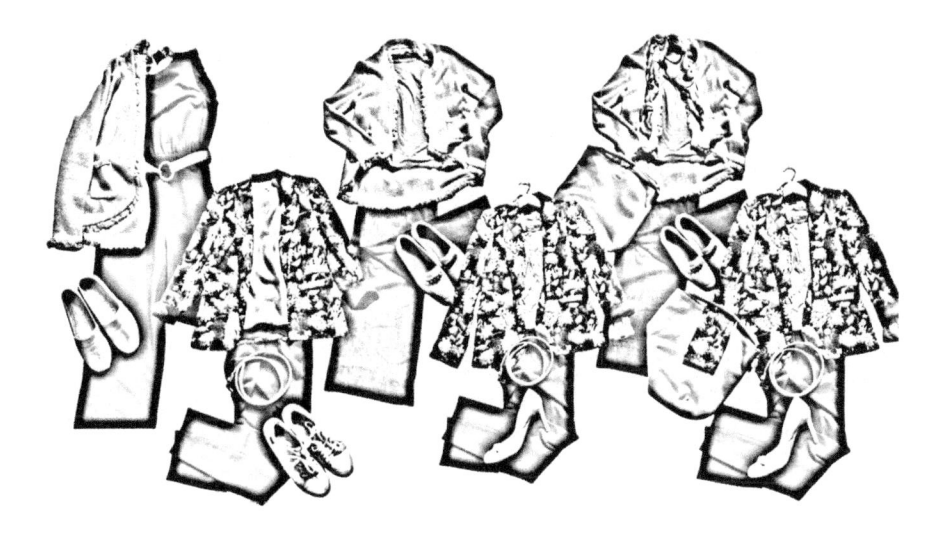

Formulate further outfit options by switching one item at a time.

Styling the Details

If your formulated outfit feels like a top and a bottom rather than a stylish curated outfit, consider what is happening between the hem of the top and the bottom half of the garment, as well as the cuffs and neckline. Exposing the cuffs, hems, and necklines of an underlayer garment adds interest and style, meaning your underlayer becomes part of the overall style – as well as being a functional layer.

Turning back cuffs and switching out an underlayer t-shirt for a blouse or shirt (underneath a sweater) adds style. You can find lots of inspiration for this on places like Pinterest, but if this sounds too fussy for your style, try sticking to one colour or tone-on-tone colour palettes. Alternatively, you could try adding a mid-layer such as a Gillet, cardi-coat, wrap, or light jacket to your outfit.

It's also useful to define what it is about your chosen garment that makes it your taste – particularly if you are not layering. For example, is it fabric, colour, print, texture, design feature, cut? What part of the outfit is the focal point? It could be the footwear or an accessory that pulls the garments together and creates your style. If so, these pieces need to be in your flat-lay photos too.

If you are going for a bold, simple style, each piece must have a defined shape.

Level Down

Continue the same process until you have sorted through all your items, creating flat-lay variables for your Level 3 outfits. Once you are satisfied with your Level 3 collection, think about levelling up or down – what can you add or lose to change from Level 3 to Level 2 or Level 4? Or even Level 5?

It might feel easier initially to Level down, but remember that even at Level 2, you will still dress as if others will see you. A casual, relaxed outfit still needs to be polished. Casual tops, t-shirts, jeans, or even joggers need to be in good condition, clean and not misshapen.

Regardless of the Level, check that your chosen outfit is a flattering look on you or be honest if you have slipped into a habit of convincing yourself it's just comfortable. Comfort alone is not enough; that's just 'making do'. You will not have an elevated wardrobe nor feel confident if you choose to 'make-do', though Level 1 Dress Code does have a place in your wardrobe.

Level Up

Upping a level to 4 and 5 will differ for everyone. You may not even have Level 5 items after your wardrobe audit. You might have a selection of 'nicer pieces' that you save for 'best', but it's my belief that there is no such thing as 'saving for best'. You should wear your best every day - because then you will feel your best every day.

Could you wear your 'nicer pieces' more?' For example, can they be styled between Levels 3 and 4? Or have you categorised them as 'special'?

Society has reached a point where we choose our own dress code – rarely can we be dressed too well, but we can easily look too sloppy. Of course, no one will tell you to your face that you look sloppy, but believe me, people do notice.

Women and men who choose to go that extra mile to ensure each outfit is thought through and the best they have never say, "I wish I chose to dress sloppier". These are the people who raise the bar for all of us and instil confidence in others to dress well.

This is definitely the case in my monthly Women's Business Network group. I always dress Level 4, and as the compliments float around the room, it's not long before others join in with a beaming smile, saying, "I love coming here because I can dress up".

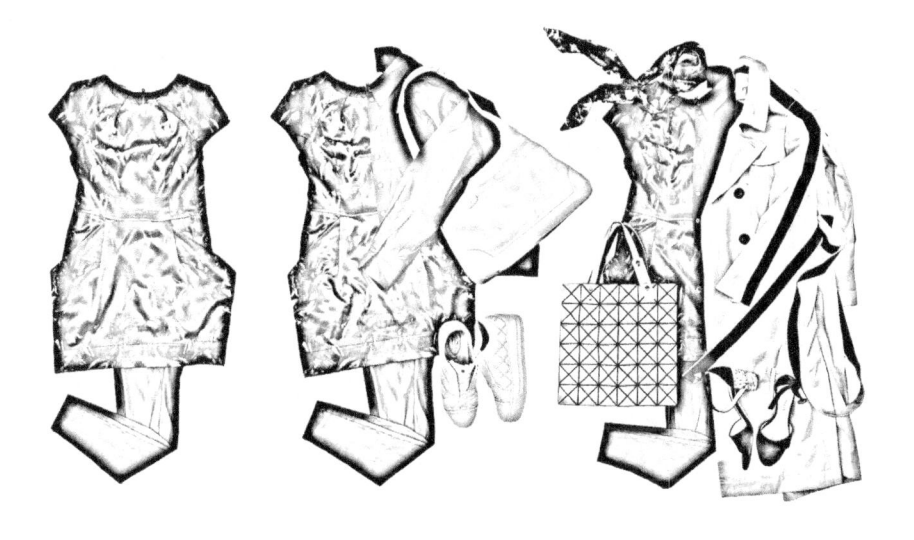

Base level 3 Dress, at home, out with a bag, level UP with coat, jewellery and heels

Dressing at Levels 3 to 4 to attend this brunch event for a duration of 90 minutes creates a genuine buzz of positivity, which we all take forward into the day ahead.

Keep Going

Now that you've mastered flat styling continue to create outfit combinations from your audited wardrobe for all Levels of your Dress Code. If you get stuck, remember to refer to your previous notes.

It is likely that you see a natural gap in your collection. Perhaps you wish you had a different pair of well-fitting dark jeans or a mid-layer jacket that is just a bit longer. At this point, you can revisit Chapter 2.2 to review the suggested list, which will help identify the garments you wish you had to formulate an outfit. Write down these items, creating a wish list of garments.

If you have odd items that don't fit into any curated outfit - what items are missing? A top, bottom, footwear, layers, accessories?

Write all of these down, too and add them to your wish list. This will be the start of your purposeful shopping list, making sourcing and shopping 'your style' so much easier.

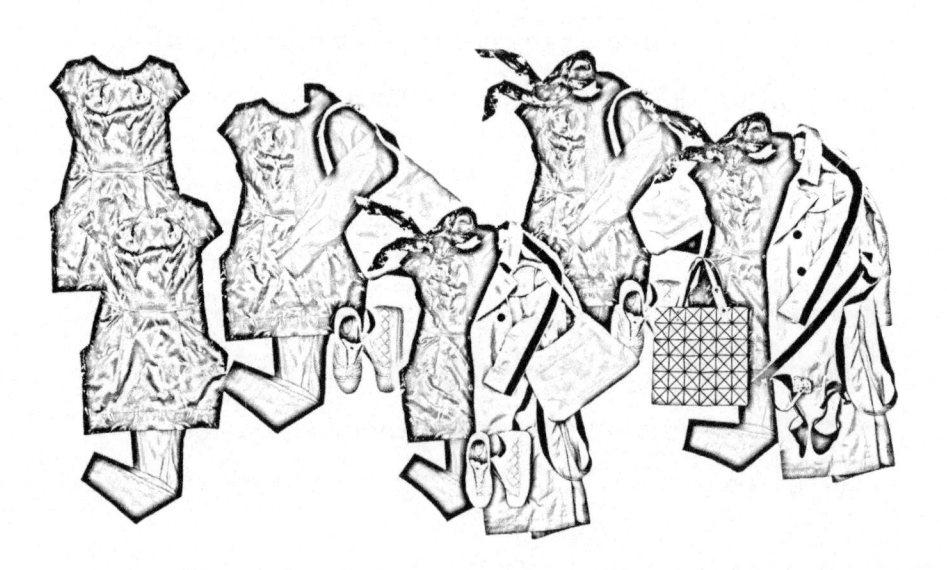

Tweak outfit options within levels, for season, day to night, and activity

How To Edit Your Clothes – Summary

- Flat laying your garments into outfits is an efficient way to formulate multiple outfit combinations quickly.
- Once you have an outfit you love, re-create it as many times as you can with to meet your Level 3 Dress Code.
- Use footwear and accessories and switch one piece at a time to style further outfits, either levelling up or down.
- Take photographs of each flat-lay outfit – even if you've only added or switched one item – so that you can log all of your looks.
- Do not try outfits on at this stage; it will take too long. From the wardrobe audit you did before editing, you know everything fits and meets your style.
- Make a note of anything missing to form your purposeful clothes shopping wish list.
- Your photographs will be a visual record of your clothes. You will be able to use these to see what works well and which tweaks you need to make to level up and down outfits.

Suggested Actions

Book out 2-hour slots in your diary to edit your clothes into flat-lays and curated outfits as soon as you can after your wardrobe audit.

Make a wish list of items you need for which outfit, plus any overall notabilities such as:

1. Do you have too many tops and not enough bottoms?
2. Do you have dresses but nothing to wear on your legs?
3. Do you favour one coat for every outfit?
4. Do you have too many Level 4/5 outfits for your current

lifestyle or vice versa?
5. Do you have a variety of shoes, and do you wear them all?

6.2 Maximising your Clothes

There is no set time for this part; simply wear and enjoy your clothes. Maximising how you wear your clothes is a matter of progression: introduce new pieces and move on from older pieces when they are no longer required. This is how you continually evolve your wardrobe and prevent yourself from getting stuck with clothes that no longer serve you.

As you wear your outfit combinations, try to remember to take an 'outfit selfie'. Outfit selfies provide the perfect image to assess how each of your new outfits looks, as well as your silhouette and proportions. This enables you to compare which clothes you love the most.

To take an outfit selfie, I have a YouTube video showing you how to set up your phone: https://www.youtube.com/watch?v=T1gWt5Ltgow. You can also ask someone in your household to take your picture or even a colleague at work.

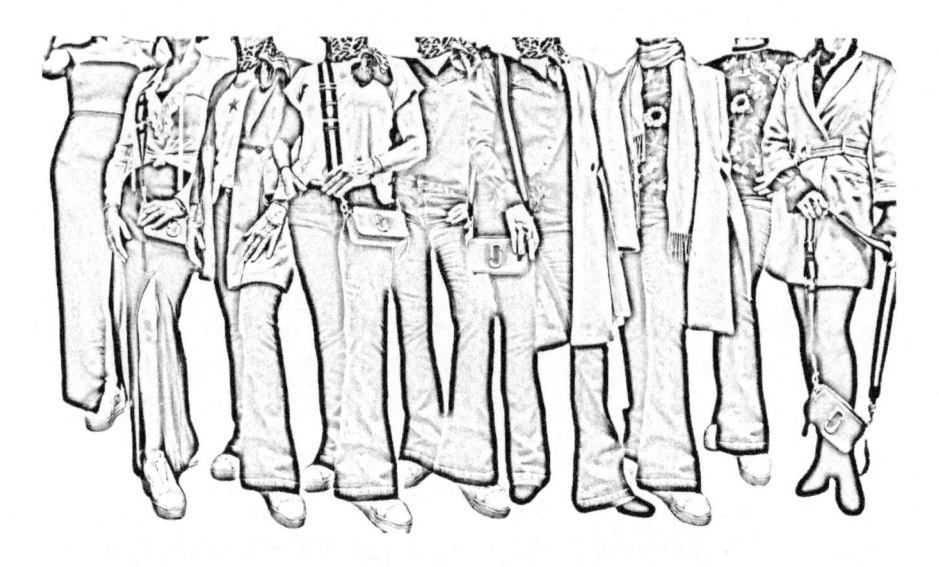

Take photos as you wear each outfit to create a log & identify your favourites.

As you make your way through your flat-styled outfits, you will discover you gravitate towards some outfits and not wear others. Keep tweaking your looks by switching pieces to make them wearable. If certain items appear in every outfit, ask yourself why. Can you pop a similar item on your wish list in a different colour or fabric to create further outfits?
Learning to maximise pieces in this way will ultimately set you in good stead, not only when it comes to investing in future buys but also knowing confidently what to wear and how this will improve your style.

If you are not wearing an outfit, try to figure out why. The most common reasons for this are:

1. You are stuck in the habit of wearing the same outfits on rotation and need a bit more confidence to wear some of your newly curated outfits. If this is the case, wear them at home first to get used to the feel. Just like a new haircut, change takes a bit of getting used to.
2. You need to go shopping. Your audit and edit have left you thread-bare, and you need to add pieces to complete your outfit edits before you can wear them. Adding more is coming up next – but as mentioned, new pieces need to be the right items if you want to improve and progress your style.

Here is an example of how just 15 items can make over 100 outfits. A great demonstration of how to maximise your clothes.

228 | 2ND SKIN

15 Items
100+ Outfits Options

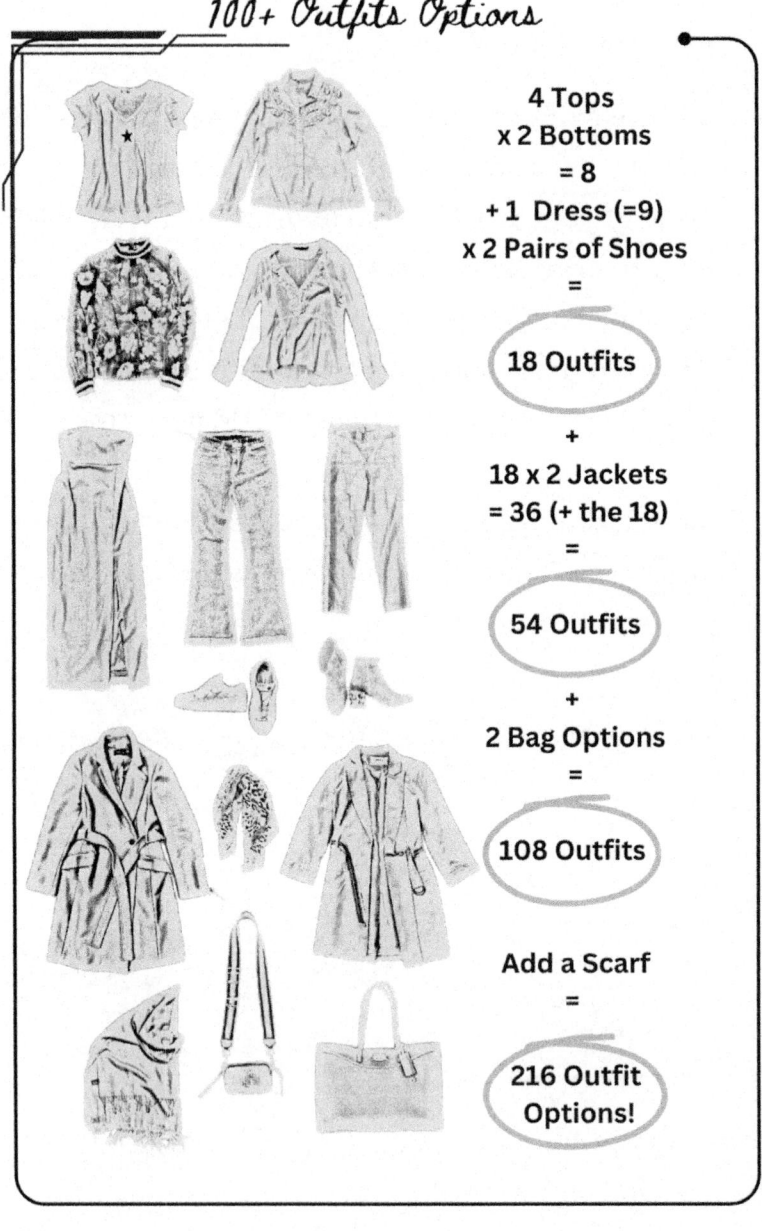

4 Tops
x 2 Bottoms
= 8
+ 1 Dress (=9)
x 2 Pairs of Shoes
=

18 Outfits

+

18 x 2 Jackets
= 36 (+ the 18)
=

54 Outfits

+

2 Bag Options
=

108 Outfits

Add a Scarf
=

216 Outfit Options!

3. There is a third possibility, too, which comes down to the success of your wardrobe audit and outfit edit.

I spoke earlier about our clothes being our closest possessions that carry memories our subconscious sometimes finds it hard to forget. This can make it difficult to see our clothes as isolated items that can be switched into a multitude of outfits because of their previous association.

Revisit Madeleine's story in Chapter 1.6, Mind Matters and then consider if you still love these items.

4. Another common reason is fear. Have you kept items that fit you, even if you don't love them because of the fear of nothing left to wear?

Revisit Angie's story in Chapter 5.3, Feeling Threadbare. Your shopping wish list is important in this scenario.

Re-style, Re-wear & Re-fashion

Don't be put off by the fact that once a garment has been seen in one scenario, you can't re-wear it and re-style it for another. You can. The truth is no one will remember, and if they do, it means they are taking notice and liking it.

A great way to re-wear outfits is when you've attended a special occasion and have bought a special outfit. Don't hide it in the wardrobe and wait for another occasion to wear it again. Use dressing down tactics, such as splitting the outfit and pairing it with Level 3 footwear and accessories or a different outer layer, to move this from a Level 5 outfit to a daily wear Level 3. This doesn't mean you can't wear it styled again for a Level 4 or 5 occasion; it's simply a great way to get value from your collection, particularly if you have some more expensive items of clothing. Also, knowing that you can re-wear and re-fashion some of your best occasion wear can help when it comes to budgeting. If you know that your outfit is not going to be a 'one wear' scenario, then you are more likely to fork out for the perfect item because, in the long run, this purchase will lead to a reduction in costs for your daily Level 3 outfits.

Sammy is one of my clients who spends on Level 3 and saves on Level 5. Sammy recently spent £240 (sale price) on a pair of Victoria Beckham jeans that she wears daily. The fit is perfect, the style is spot on, and she pairs them with an array of blouses and heels (yes, you heard correctly, heels), and they are her staple, signature look that, by her admission, she lives in. By contrast, when she was invited to a close friend's cocktail party, she bought a £35 dress from Depop, wore it again out for dinner with her partner and then two weeks later re-sold it for £40.

Always assess wearability against your lifestyle. I see so many wardrobes that contain beautiful pieces taking up wardrobe space, not being worn because the owner considers them Level 4 Dress Code and above. Instead, they spend time and money on mediocre Level 3 clothes before calling me to say they've lost their way with style and feel frumpy. Wear your stylish clothes as much as possible, and it will become a habit. Buy items that will pair with Level 4 items to re-style them down for Level 3.

Footwear

Don't underestimate the power of footwear. What you put on your feet can literally change your height, posture and look. A clean white sneaker is acceptable with almost any outfit; however, switching out for a nude heel or ankle boot will change the look. If switching from flats to a heel or flat-forms, re-assess your coat length to balance your silhouette.

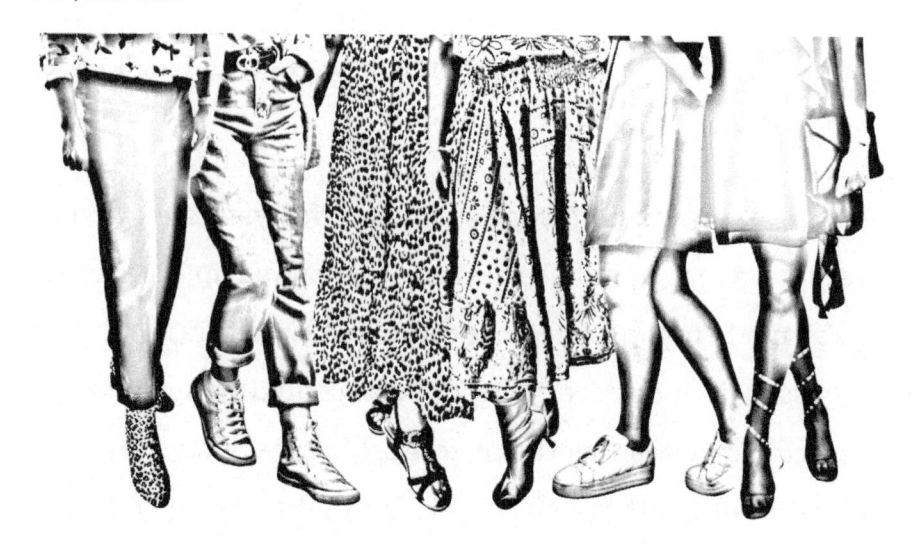

Choice of footwear alters your height, silhouette and level of dress code.

Level 5 Dress Code can be the trickiest. High-end occasions often require something new. As already mentioned throughout this book, sustainable fashion and pre-loved are big trends right now, even becoming the most popular theme of Dress Code at prestigious events. The 2020 Oscars saw the likes of Elizabeth Banks wearing a Badgley Mischka dress. Roll back 16 years, and the same dress, minus the jewelled backstrap, was her choice at the Vanity Fair Oscars Party. Adding a trim detail is an easy way to re-fashion an already-worn Level 5 outfit. Then simply pair it with different shoes and handbags.

Jane Fonda, a star known for her lifelong activism, wore the same Elie Saab gown to present the Best Picture award at the

2024 Oscars, that she first wore to the Cannes Film Festival in 2014.

Cheltenham's famous Gold Cup races took on a sustainable theme for the first time this year (2024). Race Days are infamous for attracting women parading their best attire in the hope of winning a prize at Ladies' Day. This year, the slogan was 'slow-fashion, fast-horses', in a nod to choosing sustainable fashion.

Pre-loved ensembles are interesting, and when you're not dictated by what's current on the high street, there is much more room for specific selection and wearing what you love. Utilising a mix of new, old, pre-loved, and much-loved items and habitually wearing your best conveys your visual story and personal style.

Maximising Your Clothes - Summary

- Outfit selfies are the best way to see your style.
- As you build up your library of looks, you will be able to compare your outfits, select which ones you like best, and remember which clothes work well together.
- You will be able to recognise how to level up and down outfits accordingly and identify any missing garments

that will formulate more outfits, thus maximising all your pieces.

Suggested Actions

Take outfit selfies of everything you wear. We will be using them later to refine your UPS and determine if a signature look is for you.

7. Evolving Your Ups

---·---

To be stylish for a lifetime, your wardrobe must evolve at the same pace as time, and you must manage your clothes to ensure they align with your body and lifestyle. Time does not stand still for anyone; even if you believe nothing has changed in your world, the world around you and the people around you, do. If you fail to acknowledge this fact and continue to wear the same clothes, you will become dated or frumpy.

The feeling of being dated or frumpy won't go away, which means it is likely to be unresolved. This leads to you becoming stuck in your ways and wardrobe, inevitably making the task of addressing what you wear into a challenge - which you can't face tackling.

The problem with this is that **we can still see you.**

Once you've taken the first step and have completed your wardrobe audit and edit, you need to repeat this process in a continual cycle. As your lifestyle changes and time moves on, so do societal expectations and trends which means that repeating the cycle of auditing and editing allows you to see old garments go and new items come in. You will then adjust your Dress Code Levels in accordance.

This cycle is known as 'evolving your UPS' (Unique Personal Style), and in this chapter, we will cover how to source and buy new pieces that will continually develop your UPS. This chapter will also teach you how to maintain your style in a manner that evolves with time, along with some further tips on how to progress your style so that you (and it!), don't fade with age

One important point to note here: The demise of 'traditional dress codes' means there is a bigger visual gap between those who do care what they wear and people who do not – because this is visible to us all. We are always seen.

> *Style is a way to say who you are without having to speak.*
>
> — Rachel Zoe

7.1 Creating a Signature Look from your UPS

Your Unique Personal Style (UPS) is the visual language I refer to as your second skin. The 'attention to detail' of how the wearer finishes the completed look makes a chosen outfit stylish or not.

The phrase 'attention to detail' sounds more complex than it is. Simply put, it means being aware of the intended finish of your overall look regardless of taste. For example, if you are a casual jeans wearer, you will already have learnt which trouser silhouette and cut enhance your figure shape; footwear depends on the length and width of the trouser hem, and your choices should be appropriate to the season and occasion.

If you like sweaters, is your chosen jumper fitted, slouch, chunky knit, or fine jersey, and does it require an underlayer?

If so, is your underlayer visible at the neckline, cuff, and hem to form an edging to your jumper? Does this remain in keeping with the overall intended silhouette and personal style?

This is what I mean by 'attention to detail'.

Remember Anna and Judi's story in Chapter 4? Two women who both favoured the same clothes, yet one was frumpy and dated and the other effortlessly stylish. The difference was in the 'attention to detail' of their finished style.

Let's get more specific about the detail of your style.

After your audit and edit sessions, you will have a bank of outfit selfies. Let's look at the results to find common links which support your UPS and could lead to a signature look.

'Common links' are elements which are noticeably consistent and can include:

- Silhouette – 1 or 2 obvious silhouettes.
- Garment Type – A particular garment that stands out as 'you'.
- Proportion – For example, longer-length tops or shorter upper body shapes.
- Fit – Snug to the body or loose, floaty shapes.
- Accessories – Statement jewellery, brooches, scarfs, hats etc.
- Unfussy – No accessories and sharp-shaped garment silhouettes.

- Bags – One go-to bag or different bags in every outfit.
- Footwear – Statement shoes or a variety of footwear.
- Colour – Limited colour palette, monochrome, tone-on-tone or bright colour.
- Pattern – Bold, big, ditsy, slogans, classic stripes, clash of patterns, etc.
- Texture – Lace, leather, suede, sequins, brocades, knits, etc.
- Drama – Asymmetric hems and necklines, fashion features or shoulder pads.

Remember: You are not committed to one style forever. We dress according to our body shape and lifestyle, and both continually change – even if only slightly.

This exercise might also identify a dressing habit that you no longer like. When I started taking pictures, I couldn't believe how bad I looked in a T-shirt and skinny jeans! See, even stylists get it wrong if we don't check silhouette, balance, and fabric.

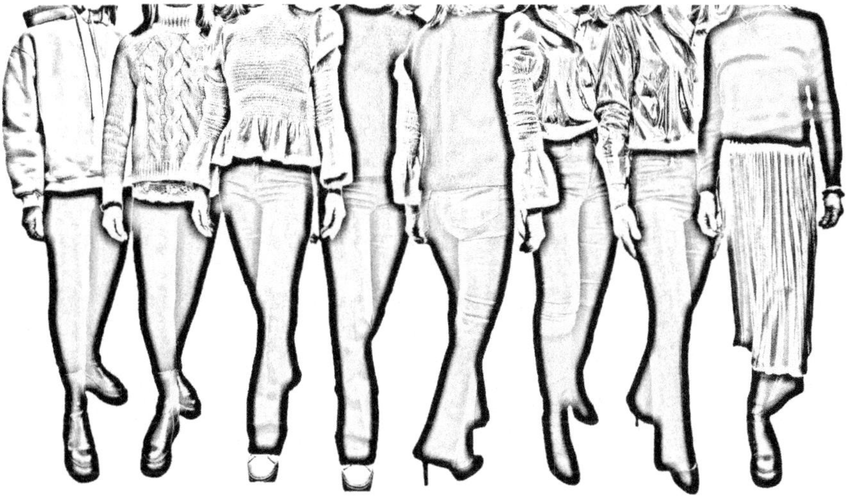

5'2" Size 06
Unique Personal Style (UPS)
Minimum colours, maximum fabric types and textures.

Image7.1

Limiting colours yet a change of footwear shifts activity, adding a layer crosses seasons, and switching to shimmery fabrics Levels UP for the evening.

From casual to polished, day to night, achieved just by switching footwear and fabric choices.

Comparing your outfits side-by-side in picture form will expose what you like the most and what you don't. Focus on what looks good and feels like you, and from this point onwards, always wear outfits that look and feel as good as your favourite ones.

Don't worry about the outfits that don't work so well; they will organically get phased out of your wardrobe through repeating the audit and edit process, and as you add fresh pieces.

By now, you should have found several or lots of outfits you love and a clearer picture of what is working for you. You may even have identified a common theme or trait that is your Signature Look.

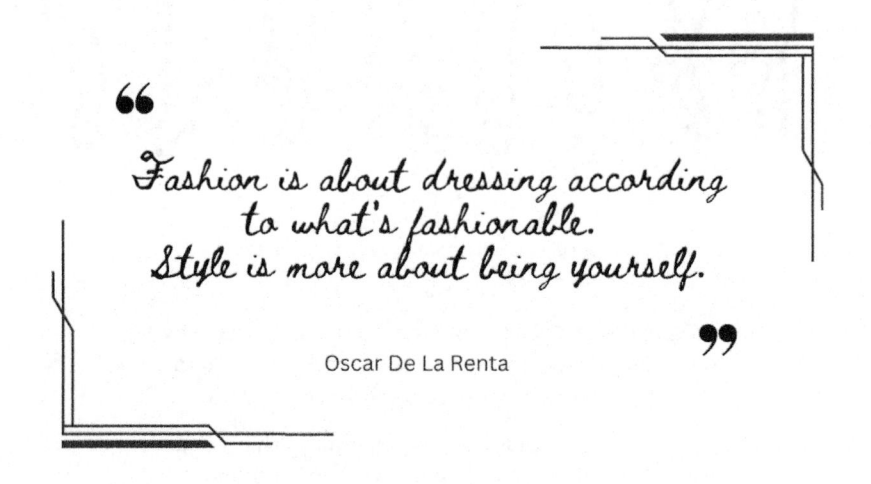

> *Fashion is about dressing according to what's fashionable. Style is more about being yourself.*
>
> Oscar De La Renta

Signature Looks

A Signature Look refers to a recurring style trait you have developed and don't want to give up. It forms your Style identity and is another layer of your UPS.

Note, though, that it is not essential to have a Signature Look. It doesn't make a person more stylish and, if not executed authentically, can even make a person look dated. You can't force it, either. A Signature Look happens over time and is a realisation that one element has remained (unintentionally) within your look for a while.

This identifying trait is usually formed over time once you are sure of your UPS and are confident you know how to evolve your silhouette with your figure and align your Dress Code Levels with your lifestyle. For example, the late Queen Elizabeth II was rarely seen wearing patterned fabrics on duty, and you'll be hard-pushed to find an image of fashion guru Trinny in a mini skirt. I recall hearing her say that she had short legs and, therefore, dressed to elongate them. These are what I mean when talking about identifying traits. You may have a signature look for your job position. Politicians tend to adhere to a consistent, expected style, a bit like a personalised uniform in a bid to represent honesty.

Signature looks can include natural assets and accessories. Dame Anna Wintour is known for her bouclé jackets and stylish dresses, but it's not her clothes per se that are her signature look; it's her sharp, thick bob and black sunglasses that make her instantly recognisable. This is probably one of the most consistent Signature Looks ever seen. You kind of expect it for the benefit of F-row fashionistas (the front row of a premier runway show), but Dame Anna still dons those blackout sunnies for an indoor TV interview at her home in the evening! That is a girl true to her Signature Look.

Another example I'd like to share is the late Steve Jobs. You only need to look back at early pictures of him to realise it took him decades to invent his black turtle neck Signature Look, and I don't doubt that a stylist had something to do with it. There is also Mark Zuckerberg's theory – as the CEO of FB serving billions of clients a day, he chooses to wear a grey t-shirt daily, claiming if he 'knows he's going to wear the same outfit' it's 'one less decision to make'.

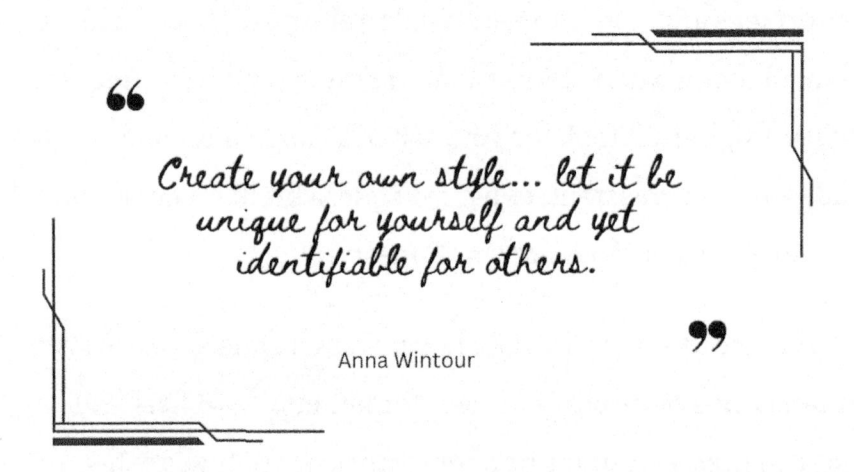

> Create your own style... let it be unique for yourself and yet identifiable for others.
>
> — Anna Wintour

Once a Signature Look is established, it can remain in place even when body shape changes. Singer Adele's Signature Look is her eyeliner (yes, make-up can be a Signature Look, too) and has remained even as her body shape has changed. As her famous natural curves disappeared, her style of fluid fabrics fitting beautifully over her bosom, nipping in under her bust and skimming over the curvature of her hips, has been replaced with clothing styles that feature peplums and flounce to add the illusion of accentuated curves to her new slimmer figure – but her eyeliner remains firmly in place.

When I was working as a lecturer, I remember one of my students asking me if I was okay. I was a little perplexed at what triggered the question and instantly wondered if I had bags under my eyes or had forgotten my blusher, but it was because I wasn't wearing a flower in my hair. My students had noticed that I wore a flower on the days they saw me, which was a detail formed from necessity and was definitely unintentional. I was a recent divorcee, working mum, dropping my two youngsters at nursery and pre-school before getting to college on time, leaving no time for hairstyling. An up-do secured by a flower clip that matched my outfit or silk neck scarf became my go-to and unknowingly was my Signature Look.

246 | 2ND SKIN

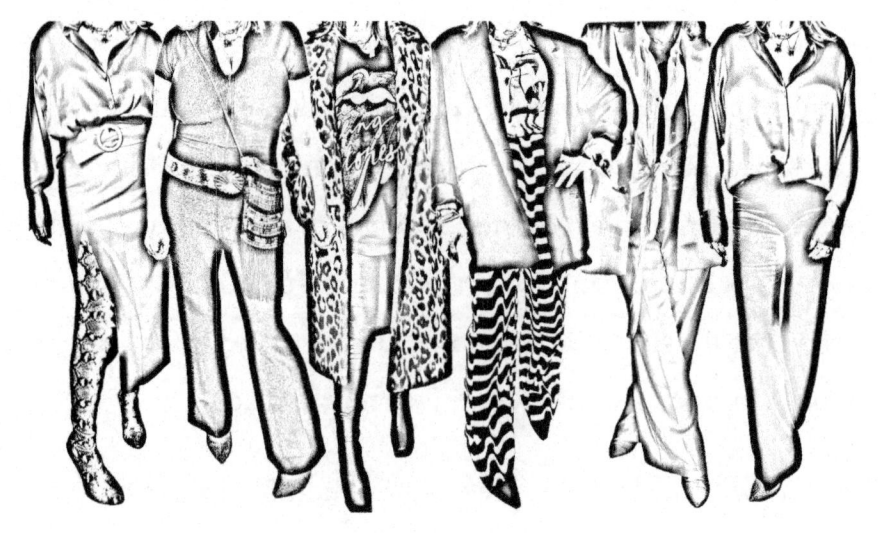

5'2" Size 14
Signature Looks

Colour & pattern first meet the senses – however, jewellery is the one consistent feature in every outfit, on every level.

From casual to polished, day to night, the same necklace appears on its own or mixed with further pieces.

Signature Look (Within Your Ups) – Summary

- Finding your UPS is recognising common links between your outfits.
- For example, this can be a colour palette, silhouette, bold pattern, or a recurring fashion feature.
- Make-up, hair, and accessories can also be part of your UPS.
- A Signature Look develops over time and can be as simple as one item that is always present in every outfit.
- It could be a specific garment, accessory, dramatic hairstyle, or lipstick that is part of every outfit, no matter what you wear, at any level of your dress code.

- A Signature Look can also be developed for certain areas of your life, not your entire life, such as just work or a particular (regular) activity.

Suggested Actions

1. Identify style consistencies and links that you notice in your Outfit Selfies.
2. Make a note of looks and traits you see that you want to move away from.
3. Do you notice any distinct styles that can be grouped together for certain aspects of your life? If yes, can this be carried through to all your looks, or is it an area of your life you want to keep as a separate dress code?

UPS Troubleshooting

?	Chapter	✓
I'm unsure what UPS or Unique Personal Style is?	Revisit Chapter 4.3 UPS Explained	This chapter explains where we are with today's dress codes.
I can't identify any consistent style links?	Revisit Chapter 3 Style Formulas	Consider the pros & cons then book a formula session if you need a boost.
All my Outfits are completely different?	Revisit Chapter 6.1 Edit Outfits	Follow the process of switching one item to create a new outfit.

Ups Troubleshooting

If you are still struggling to define your UPS, it might be because your clothes aren't feeling right. You can follow all the advice in the world about what looks good on you (and you are following advice right now by getting this far through 2nd SKIN!); however, your outfits still need to feel right.

If this resonates, revisit Chapter 1 and review the answers you gave under Suggested Actions. Perhaps pick an outfit from your style history that you loved because it made you feel so happy when you wore it. Don't describe the garments;

describe why that outfit felt special. Was it because it gave you confidence? Was it because it fitted your life as it was then? Is it because it perfectly represented how you wanted to be seen by your peers? The idea is to reignite that same feeling of excitement and confidence with what you choose to wear today.

7.2 Finding STYLE Inspiration

Inspiration comes from the World around us in the form of what we see, hear, smell, touch, and taste. Our senses notice, pick up and respond to different stimulants in varying amounts.

It's the same with clothing. You look for, or subconsciously notice, things that stir your senses. When that sense is a feeling of enthusiasm, it is a new and creative idea, and you have found inspiration - otherwise known as Style Inspo.

The saturated fashion market has sometimes made clothing-related inspiration blur into one. The principles required to navigate saturation and evolve your style are learning to see through the noise and the blur and focusing only on what you are attracted to and what has a potential purpose within your clothes collection.

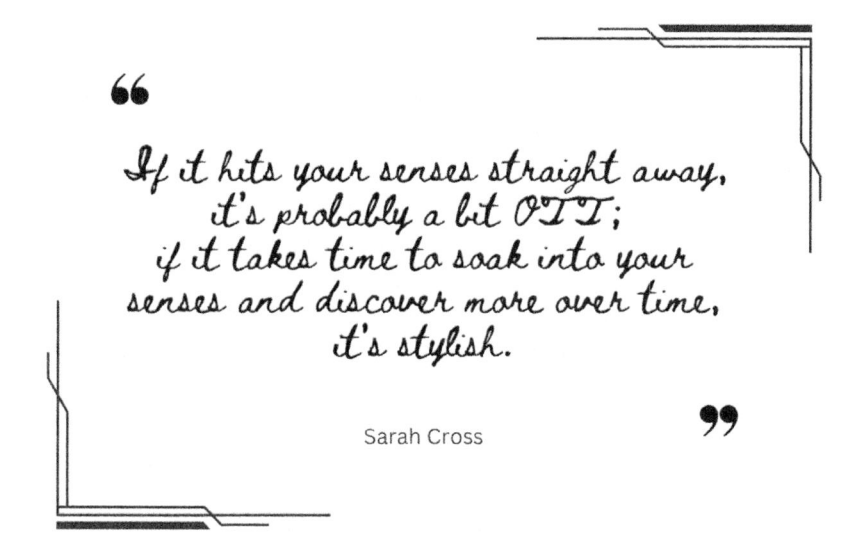

> *If it hits your senses straight away, it's probably a bit OTT; if it takes time to soak into your senses and discover more over time, it's stylish.*
>
> Sarah Cross

When it comes to dressing, there are two main sources of inspiration:

1. Clothes themselves
2. How other people and influencers wear clothes

Influencer Inspiration

This is a method of identifying a person or a few people you identify with because they represent you in some way. They could have a similar body shape to you, similar interests to you, frequent the types of places you like to go, are in the same age bracket as you, have the same taste, or showcase a lifestyle you aspire to. Their life resonates with you, so how they dress could align with your lifestyle, body or how you see your life in the future.

Instagram

Thanks to Instagram (or IG), here's a process of finding them:

> Note: You need an Instagram profile to search and view, but you can use any nickname and don't need to upload content. You can browse and follow without revealing anything about yourself unless you want to. It is free and worth having the app.

- Start with a celebrity or influencer you are already a fan of – a known style icon, model, someone you've seen on TV or in a magazine feature, heard on a podcast or radio, an actress, a singer, an A-lister or a Z-lister. Anyone.
- Find them on Instagram and follow them. This will give you a first look at what they wear, how they style their looks, and some ideas that you could implement into your style.
- But it's the next layer that will provide untapped inspiration – and that layer is the other people who follow them. Scroll down their followers list to see people who are also fans of your celebrity person.
- Within their fanbase, you will find influencers, fashion bloggers and normal people who will already be taking inspiration from your celebrity and showcasing it on their IG profiles.
- These fans provide a ready-made bank of outfit ideas inspired by your stylish icon, in a way that might resonate with you more or directly align to your

lifestyle.
- You can also look at who your stylish celebrity is getting their inspiration from by scrolling through who they follow.

For example, @erica_Davies is a curvy size 14, aged 46, married with two kids, and typically wears bright colours, bold prints, floaty dresses, drawstring pants, t-shirts, jumpsuits, and blazers. Erica is a fashion writer, so this is a good starting point if her profile resonates with you or if you are new to IG and want to follow this example.

If you look at who Erica follows, you will see that there is a full mix:

- @thecreativeclassicist showcases a page of plain, neutral separates with a formal edge; not a single bold pattern is to be seen here.
- @myenglishcountrycottage showcases a feminine, bohemian country look and has dedicated 'story highlights' of her fashion looks.
- @stylebynanny, who claims to break the fashion rules, has story highlights for each season.

If any of those sound more like your style, check them out and see who follows them.

Other Social Media

If you're still unsure where to start and the only celebrities you can think of are fashionista-stylist types you do not identify with, try a Google search for someone in your field. For example, if you are a female gardener in the UK, you could search for famous female gardeners UK, which will bring up names and images and their IG account if they have one.

Once you have found one, just look at both their followers and who they follow.

Social media is an open door to non-celebrities, too, and there are thousands of women, just like you, showing off great looks and showcasing ideas that you will find inspirational and easy to replicate in your style.

If you are still wondering where to start, ask your Facebook community which IG accounts they suggest are good for style inspiration.

Alternatively, if you don't want a Facebook account or any of the other social media platforms, you can still find more than enough inspiration with a Google (or similar) search, as suggested above.

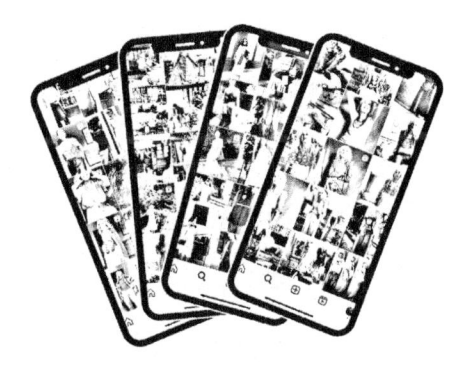

Instagram is a great place for style inspiration

Clothing Inspiration

Unlike influencer inspiration, which showcases lifestyle scenarios (to influence your feelings about outfits, amongst other things), clothing inspiration relates specifically to garments which catch your senses.

Here are three ways you capture clothing inspiration:

1. ACCIDENTAL When you're not actively looking for clothing inspiration but as you go about your daily business, your senses are agitated by what someone is wearing. It could be a person on the street, at work, a picture in a leaflet, or on a billboard.

2. ACTIVELY When you are on a mission to find clothes, you can go clothes shopping, scroll through clothing brands online, Google clothing items, or subscribe to style mailing lists, blogs, or personalised garment distributors.

3. THE EXPOSURE EFFECT Clothing that has deliberately been put in front of your senses, albeit by algorithms. This includes non-clothing marketing campaigns like lifestyle products, cars, holidays, perfumes, and drinks, clothing brand sponsorships, and general market saturations via any means.

A well-known selling concept states that if someone has seen, heard or encountered something approximately 27 times, the brain finds the familiarity comforting – potentially leading to purchase.

When we're learning about something we're interested in, it's a natural human response to build trust the more we are exposed to it. This is great if the product we are exposed to is something we need and want, but it's often why I find wardrobes full of unsuitable items. Our senses saw them enough to believe they were the items we were expected to have. It's how I - and many others - ended up wearing skinny jeans even though the silhouette only suits a few figure types.

How to Interpret Style Inspiration

Now you know how to find inspiration; interpreting it into outfits doesn't always mean a like-for-like copy.

Notice I used the term outfits. If you are inspired to source one garment like-for-like, it still needs to be put into an outfit, which will be based on your interpretation.

The easiest way to do this is to use the editing process in Chapter 6 and swap out a garment from one of your ready-to-wear looks for your new one. Check out your outfit selfie bank, too. If your inspiration piece is a dress, would the footwear and outerwear you already style with your existing dresses work with the new one? The same goes for a coat, etc.

Influencer inspiration, which is usually completed outfits, will have specific traits that stir your senses. Look deeper than just colour, pattern, and shape and identify details and finishes. Often, it is something you've seen before or a reminder of something you used to own and wear. Pinpoint what you like best about the inspirational outfit, and if it is wildly different to what you usually wear, use Pinterest, for example, or an internet search to look at more similar outfits.

If you're unfamiliar with Pinterest, it is an app described as a 'visual discovery engine for finding ideas including style inspiration'. It allows you to 'pin' images and group them together for easy reference. This is technically another source of inspiration; however, Pinterest (like much of today's social media) is full of fashion marketing noise and sponsored ads, making it easy to get distracted and lose focus on what you are looking for.

Once you are at the stage of interpreting inspiration, Pinterest is great because you can be specific with your search for garments and looks and find a range of ideas closest to your UPS. These ideas will then be easier to interpret into your wardrobe.

For example, you can search for loose-fit summer pants or chunky knit scarf outfits and add style words like classic blazers for women or comfortable chic outfits. As I've already said, this tool is best used after you have established your UPS and dress code to ensure you have a reason and direction for your search.

Sally loved the look of the big chunky scarf and excitedly bought one. She didn't know how to wear it well because she assumed it was a high winter item and tried to pair it with her winter coats. It didn't work; it just looked bulky and uncomfortable. The scarf was a statement piece and needed to be the focal point of her outfit. To explain this to Sally, I found images on Pinterest showing her options that she could choose to fit her style. This meant she could enjoy wearing the scarf she had been so happy to purchase.

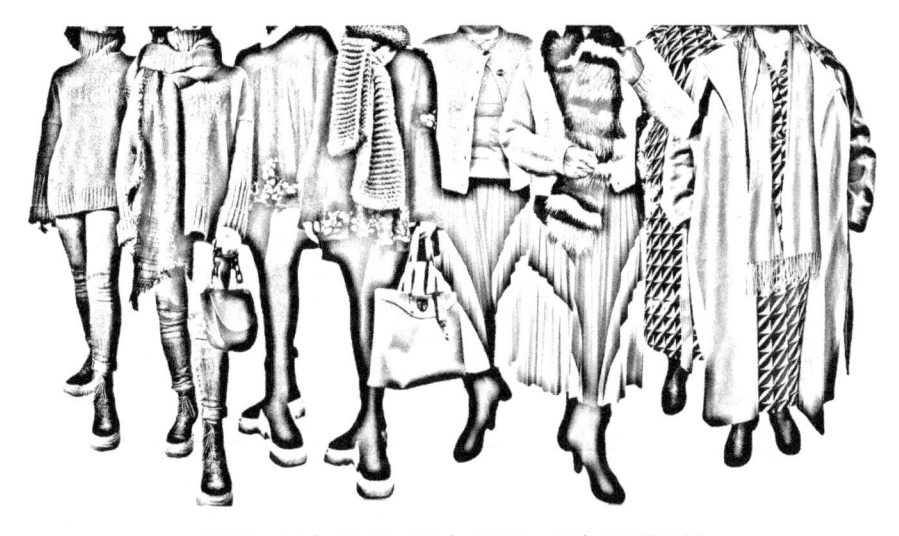

5'0" Size 08 | 5'6" Size 12 | 5'3" Size 14 | 5'5" Size 22

Use Inspiration to add or refine elements of your Outfit,
rather than copying an entire look
These 4 examples show how a feature scarf can personalise an Outfit

Another example is the Bohemian feminine look, which is pretty and attractive yet often pictured as a summer look. Darker base colours, though, can make the look seasonless and be styled with leather or pleather outerwear, warm tights, an oversized handbag and boots.

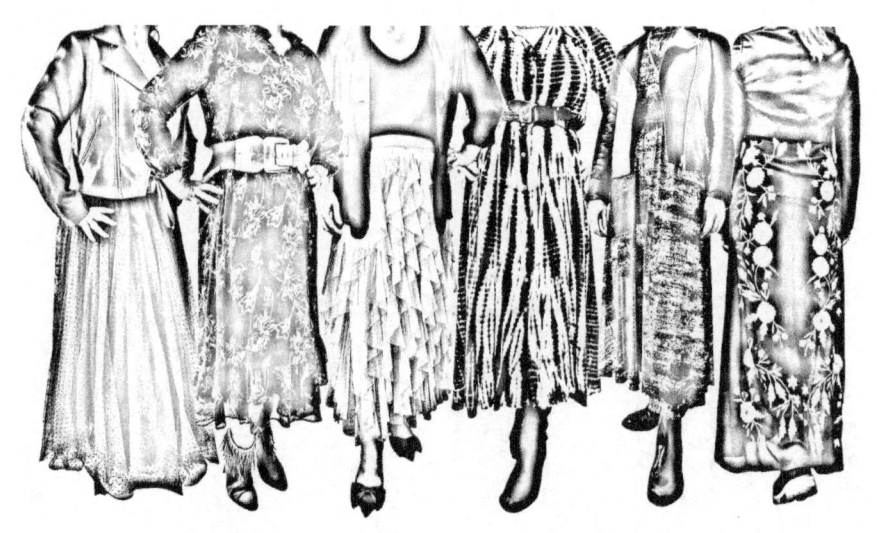

5'5" Size 14 | 5'5" Size 14 | 5'9" Size 16 | 5'6" Size 16 | 5'0" Size 08 | 5'6" Size 12

Use Inspiration to Style Your Clothes for all Seasons
Summer Boho pieces can be styled with leather
jackets & Boots for all seasons.

If your inspiration is a completely new look that you want to experiment with, do it. If it works and is as good as or better than your current favourite outfits, use this new outfit as your starter for further editing as you progress your wardrobe through your lifetime.

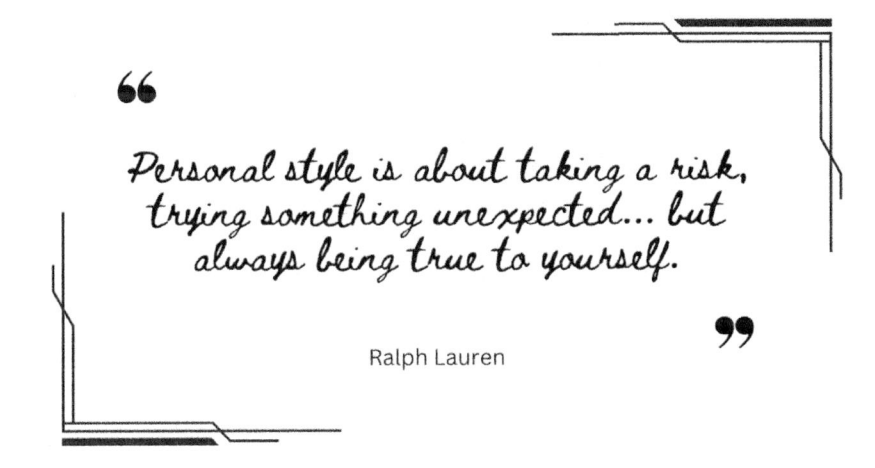

> *Personal style is about taking a risk, trying something unexpected... but always being true to yourself.*
>
> Ralph Lauren

Style Inspiration - Summary

- Style Inspiration is seeing a look or a piece of clothing that excites you.
- Wearing it or implementing it in your wardrobe should make you feel as good as the excitement you experienced when you first saw it.
- Use both influencer and clothing inspiration to add ideas, update outfits and continually progress your wardrobe looks.
- Use your outfit selfies to switch out new garments to ensure you have something to wear with your new pieces.
- Use Pinterest to learn how your inspiration can stay true to your UPS, dress code and align with your current lifestyle.

Suggested Actions

If you haven't already got an Instagram account open one. You can set it as private and use it to find style inspiration without having to upload any content yourself.

Find three celebs that you resonate with. Here are a few suggestions to start your search:

@erica_davies @carla.rockmore @emmahill @tamumcpherson @iconaccidental @Trinnywoodall @funmiford @seasonsofella @jessontheplussize @thecreativeclassicist @myenglishcountrycottage @stylebynanny

Do the same with Pinterest. Start by making a pin board of styles seen on your Instagram influencers.

Other Options:
    Subscribe to a style newsletter.
    Follow fashion bloggers or store blogs.
    Read magazines or style supplements.

I don't recommend signing up for all these options because you would be back at saturation point. Just choose the platform or newsletter/blog you enjoy most, then switch to another if it isn't giving you the inspiration you want.

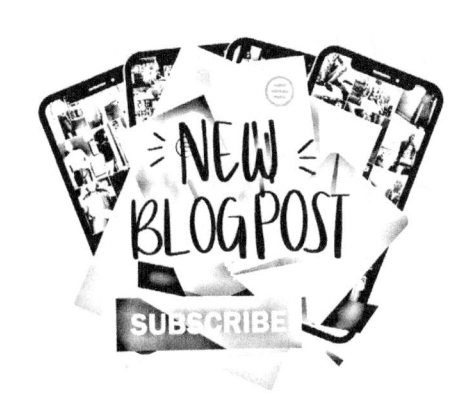

7.3 Shopping & Sourcing Guide

From this point onwards, you do not need to guess, make do, or accept any clothes or wardrobe items that are not your UPS or don't align with your lifestyle.

Shopping is a hobby for some, a chore for others, and a skill that needs mastering for the time-poor. Either way, it's certainly more beneficial to your style and wardrobe management if you have your shopping list to hand – comprised partly of the missing key items you identified during your wardrobe edit in Chapter 6, plus pieces from your newfound inspiration.

Just like dress codes, the way we shop has evolved, too. When I first started clothes shopping, it was an hour's bus ride to the city centre of Bristol or a day trip on the train to Birmingham, followed by trawling the stores until my feet couldn't carry me any further. This was in addition to flicking through my mum's bi-annual Marshall Ward catalogue. During this time, I never heard a single complaint about being unable to find clothes.

The high street changed when George Davies launched NEXT. It was the first store that helped women dress from outfit suggestions, like in catalogues, but in a real-life experience. To this day, the clothes are displayed in outfit suggestions rather than as single pieces. Jackets on the top rail, skirts and trousers on the bottom and a free-standing rail of several different top options that all mix and match to make up a finished curated outfit of your choice. For a short time, NEXT revolutionised the catalogue experience, too, adding real touchable fabric samples. I remember the hype and the second wave of hype when the hardback, fabric-swatched catalogues were no longer a freebie. If you don't mind the catalogue look, the formula worked well for many and still does today.

Roll on 35 years, and we have had over two decades of online shopping, which lets us view clothes in a matter of seconds from nearly anywhere in the World - all without stepping a foot outside.

In addition to online clothes shopping, there are pre-loved and pre-order offerings, which make clothing available at every price point. You'd think the wider choice would make it easier to find your perfect clothes – well, the good news is, it has.

Your dream clothes are literally at your fingertips; they are just hidden amidst the colossal mass of clothing shopping choices.

Let's go and find them.

Treat Clothes Shopping like an Audition
Preparing before shopping will give you a much higher success rate and make the experience enjoyable. It also helps with time management. I know this because when I shop for clients, I work within the time quota they are paying me for and produce the results they are expecting within their budget. I even find things in the same shops my clients claim they have already looked in. The difference is that I prepare by making a plan, and that's what I'm going to share with you now.

To make your plan, there are two essential pieces of information you need:

1. Budget
2. Purposeful shopping list

These 2 pieces of information ultimately focus your search, saving you time and increasing the success rate of purchases. Your allowance determines the budget, and your purposeful shopping is based on the list you've been making during your editing sessions and what you need for your current lifestyle. If you haven't made a shopping list, go back through Wardrobe Therapy Chapters 5 and 6 and review your notes in the Suggested Activities.

The items on your shopping list can be found online or in person. If you don't have any restrictions or reasons preventing you from doing so, I recommend combining both. Both are suitable for any budget, with brand-new and pre-loved available.

In-Store Clothes Shopping NEW

What are you going to wear?

It's a serious question. You only want purchases that will make you look and feel as good as, or better than, your best look. So, wear your best outfit when you go shopping to set the expectation and prevent you from settling for a purchase that isn't right. When you look in the changing rooms with full-length mirrors, complete with back and side angles, you want to feel good.

You have your shopping list; don't stray from it. If it's a long list, you will need to break it down, starting with what is essential first. Which one piece will make the biggest difference to you and your outfit creations? Avoid trying to look for everything in one go; it'll take too long and distract you from finding the perfect 10 out of 10 pieces.

As soon as you find your piece, it must be a 'YES' to the same questions you asked during your wardrobe audit:

1. Does the garment fit you today?
2. Do you love it 100%, and does it make you feel good when you put it on?

You don't need question 3 because in-store purchases are in excellent condition.

Buy it as soon as you find it. If you think something better might be in the next store, that indicates it's not 10 out of 10. If a better item is found later, return the first one immediately. It's no extra walking distance than if you hadn't bought it and needed to return it after checking more stores. Alternatively, consider if both pieces are perfect and align with your outfit combinations in your wardrobe. If yes, buy both. Wear one, and don't remove the tags until you've worn the first several times. If you don't reach for the second one, take it back. You've then learnt that buying twice isn't right for you and you won't do it again. Or you will have made the right decision and have more outfits you love.

Department stores make it easier to look, compare, and take several items into the changing room. It's a good idea to take a couple of sizes to try, even if the garment count is limited in the changing area. The assistant will hold the size variants for you and swap the items with you as you try them on.

Independent Boutiques are limited by style and price point, so they are easy to rule in or out depending on your budget boundaries and UPS. However, I do recommend trying these. If you have your shopping list, the shop assistants will be able to guide you easily and quickly, and they will be experts in picking out your size, too.

Take a friend. A second opinion can be useful, but be sure to let them know what you are looking for. Remember, they are there to help and support you but if they are also shopping, and are more confident with their body and look, and have a bigger budget than you, it could be more off-putting than helpful.

A quick note about fit:

Hems can be taken up and seams adjusted. Check if the store offers this service, or revisit Chapter 2.3 for a reminder of how to get alterations done.

In-Store Clothes Shopping Pre-Loved

It is essentially the same as how you shop in-store for new clothes but without the range of sizes in each style. Each piece is effectively a 'one-off' and the store layout will have its own system of how the items are filed for display. Navigating this type of store is much quicker because you are directed to your size and garment type immediately.

A typical system in a charity/thrift/opt shop is clothes sorted into garment type and size. For example, dresses, tops, skirts, trousers, and coats, followed by sizes they have, from smallest to largest. You know what garment type you are shopping for because it's on your list, so go to that section, scan the rail for the sizing information, which is usually clearly marked on the hook of the hanger, and only look there. Some have a 'designer' rail which contains higher-end labels. If the order of clothes displayed is not obvious, ask the shop assistant.

Vintage stores use a system where they display clothes from

a certain era or iconic style together. Some have an in-house seamstress who will make 'fit alterations' on purchases while you wait.

Dress Agencies sell pre-loved on behalf of individual owners, taking up to 70% of the price tag to cover costs and make their profit. They tend to mostly take high-end brands, and all pieces are fully inspected for condition. To make the experience even more appealing the stores are merchandised to look like designer Boutiques by displaying clothes by colour code and rotating stock according to season, and annual themes.

To get the full experience of pre-loved stores, I recommend you introduce yourself to the staff and let them know what you are looking for. They might have something stashed away in the storeroom just for you. Furthermore, if you are looking for specifics, which you are because you have a shopping list, Dress Agencies are usually happy to take your number and call you if something comes in. It's a good idea to take them up on this offer because when you have a surplus to move on in the future, you can sell at the same agency you buy from.

A quick note about size labels & condition:

- If you are switching from low-cost fast fashion to pre-

loved, consider the next size up. A lot of garments that are high-end brands, Vintage or Italian come up slightly smaller.
- The items have been previously worn or stored in places other than the expected manufacture-to-consumer storage. This means you need to ask all three audit questions before purchasing:

1. Does the garment fit you today?
2. Do you love it 100%, and it makes you feel good when you put it on?
3. Is the garment in excellent condition without the need for repair or alteration?

Online Clothes Shopping NEW

We live in an omni-channel society, where the integration of online, offline, AI and personalised experience is the norm for retail. This seamless approach of receiving an SMS while in-store browsing, an email reminder that you have left something in your shopping cart, or even adding another suggested item into your shopping cart with a note saying 'selected just for you' is all about wooing you into spending more. And it works. Technology and automation collate your viewing habits at an astounding rate, processing the data and feeding it straight back to you, telling you what you like and making it 'easy' for you to buy more. It's not a coincidence that a fashion advert pops up on FB when scrolling through our friends' holiday snaps.

Just like when you're looking for inspiration, do not be swayed by the power of marketing strategies that keep showing you the same thing until you give in and buy. Stick with your shopping list.

To find your shopping list items online, start with a general Google search and type in the description of the garment you are looking for, followed by the word shopping. For example, 'Green Coat Shopping'.

The result will be endless options, including what you are looking for, followed by disappointment. You've seen your perfect shopping list item, but it's out-of-stock, last season, not your size, and not shipped to your country... whatever the reason, you can't have it after all.

This *will* happen with online shopping; however, try not to be disheartened. Use the filters to add your size and country for delivery. If the item is being sold through a distribution marketplace, do another search directly on the brand's website.

When you do find your item and before buying it, do some further checks around the site. Check where they are delivering from, their returns policy, how you can contact them, what their privacy policy is, and if they have an 'about' page where you can check the seller's integrity and values. This should all be easy to find, and if not, or you have found a bargain that is too good to be true – your suspicions will probably be right. Don't buy.

Established stores like John Lewis, Selfridges or NEXT have oodles of options and sell lots of different brands. They have search filters for type, occasion, size, price, colour, and brand. You have the option to collect from the store or a pick-up point. When your package arrives, try it straight away for fit and ask the questions:

1. Does the garment fit you today?
2. Do you love it 100%, and does it make you feel good when you put it on?

If it's a no, package it up back in the original packaging and don't delay the return.

Online Clothes Shopping Pre-loved

Start your search directly on a pre-loved app or online marketplace. Chapter 5.4 lists a few of them. Usually, you will buy from the same apps and sites you use to sell your pre-loved, surplus items.

Similar to shopping pre-loved in-store, items sold online are 'one-offs,' so the only way for consumers to find anything is via search filters.

The filters are super effective, and in addition to size include condition, colour, fabric, style, price point, brand, new with tags, and new without tags. Any flaws will be mentioned in the product description and might not be visible in the photo so do check.

The same rules apply to all the other shopping sources. As soon as you receive your pre-loved item, ask the same questions you asked during your wardrobe audit:

1. Does the garment fit you today?
2. Do you love it 100%, and it makes you feel good when you put it on?
3. Is the garment in excellent condition without the need for repair or alteration?

If an item is not in mint condition, it will be detailed in the description or shown in the photos. If it wasn't you will be able to claim a refund. The same applies if an item is counterfeit. This doesn't happen often, but if you're worried, there is an option to message the seller and ask before you buy. You can also ask the seller any questions before you buy, including measurements of the garment.

It is not a standard policy to return pre-loved clothes and wardrobe items. If they don't fit, could seamstress attention be an option? Or you will need to re-sell or donate so as not to clutter up your audited wardrobe.

The non-returns policy is the trade-in for lower-priced yet quality items.

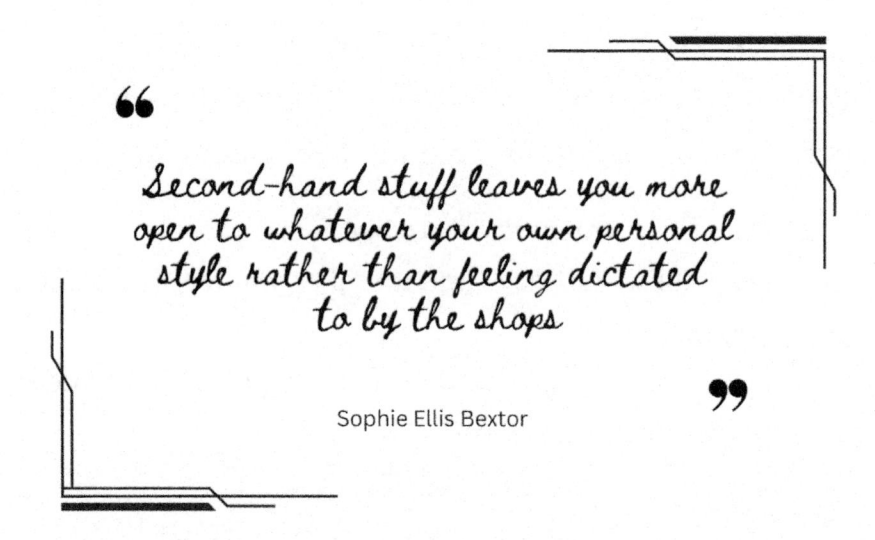

> *Second-hand stuff leaves you more open to whatever your own personal style rather than feeling dictated to by the shops*
>
> — Sophie Ellis Bextor

Budget

There are enough garments already in existence to clothe the next seven generations. However, more clothes, including fast fashion and ultra-fast fashion, are being made.

Couple this fact with the growing pre-loved market, and clothes are more affordable now than ever before in history. The pre-loved market not only provides high-end pieces at budget-friendly prices, but it is also sustainable, more ethical, circular, and a method of monetising your surplus items as explained in Chapter 5, What to do with surplus clothes.

Many of my budget-conscious clients who follow my audit, edit, and shopping list system reassess their budget once they know they are buying clothes they love to wear. Price per piece doubles and triples, yet savings are made by maximising outfit combinations and wear, making further savings on buying less. Panic buys and subpar purchases are thus reduced.

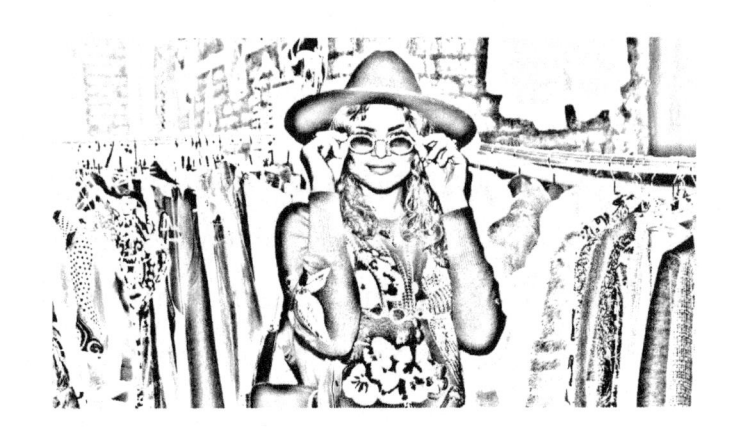

7.4 FADS, TRENDS & when to Invest

Fads last from a season to a year. They are easy to spot because they come and go quickly enough that if it didn't excite your senses, you didn't go for it. Pumpkin orange is a typical example of a *fad* colour. Not everyone's cup of tea, but those who love it are excited to see it, buy it and enjoy wearing it.

Skinnies (skinny jeans), on the other hand, started as a *fad* and became a trend. A *trend* lasts 4 to 5 years, and when the skinnies fad developed into a trend, women and men who did not suit them started buying and wearing them even though they give the illusion of adding 5lbs to your weight and show unsightly crotch bulges front and back. They really only suit a straight figure, a confident curvy figure with a flat stomach and small waist, or women with larger middles but good long legs if worn with a loose top.

Just because a fad becomes a trend, if it's not right for your body type, avoid it. When a new fad does come out, be patient and wait for it to develop. You'll see all the variations and price points as time goes on, and then you can opt-in when and if it becomes your style.

Invest in pieces that are 100% perfect and cannot be replicated. For example, wow pieces that can be worn often and across seasons, like a handbag, scarf, jacket, coat, Level 3 trousers, and jeans. Spend on items that are hard to find, for example, jeans that fit perfectly and items you want to wear daily. Shapewear, shoes, hair care, and skin care are all part of your daily look and should feel worth the spend, too.

Save on pieces you know are easy to find and fit you. Textured clothing can look chic and can be inexpensive, and if you mix high-end, medium and low-end brands, it creates the best personal style. If everything you wear is cheap, you will look cheap, and if everything you buy is expensive, the excitement of specialness fades.

Clothes shopping is traditionally segregated into menswear and womenswear, but there's a growing trend towards gender-neutral and inclusive fashion lines. Gender still plays a significant role in how clothing brands target their market, though, so you may need to adjust your search.

A 'timeless' piece never dates and is often jewellery or an item that forms a Signature Look. They are pieces that only you can discover as your UPS evolves – you won't have them on a list to pick from. More about this coming up in Chapter 8 - Finishing Touches.

Clothes Shopping - Summary

- Successful clothes shopping, whether in-person or online, starts with your purposeful shopping list, which you create while editing outfits from your wardrobe.
- This list needs to align your clothing needs with your current lifestyle.
- As your lifestyle and body shape change and your taste in clothes develop, ideas from your sources of inspiration will also then need to be added to your shopping list in order to progress your UPS.
- Clothing is more accessible and affordable than ever before.
- The growing pre-loved market is making a huge impact on pricing, quality, and choice. People are becoming well-informed about global trends and sustainability issues, and their wardrobe choices reflect that awareness, too.
- Sometimes, you might see something and instantly fall in love with it. If you have that strong desire, then buy

it, but be sure to formulate it into an outfit straight away and wear it. Don't wait.

Suggested Actions

Plan your clothes shopping. If in person, plan your best outfit to wear whilst you are shopping, including suitable footwear and appropriate shaping underwear.

Before Shopping checklist:

1. Your shopping list – items identified from your wardrobe edit and inspiration.
2. In-store shopping – a plan of which shops and your route.
3. Limit to a maximum of 5 items in any one shopping session.
4. Online shopping – use as many search filters as available to you.

During:

1. Don't buy when bored, scrolling, or after a few glasses of wine!

After shopping checklist:

1. Try on and if not 10 out of 10 return items straight

away.

2. Curate your new items into outfits and wear them ASAP

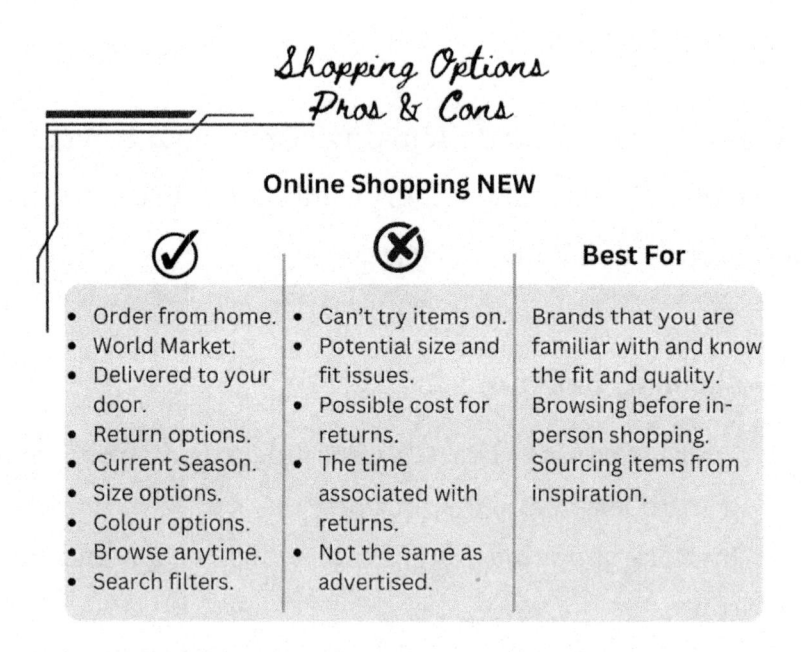

Shopping Options Pros & Cons

Online Shopping NEW

✓	✗	Best For
- Order from home. - World Market. - Delivered to your door. - Return options. - Current Season. - Size options. - Colour options. - Browse anytime. - Search filters.	- Can't try items on. - Potential size and fit issues. - Possible cost for returns. - The time associated with returns. - Not the same as advertised.	Brands that you are familiar with and know the fit and quality. Browsing before in-person shopping. Sourcing items from inspiration.

Online Shopping PRE-LOVED

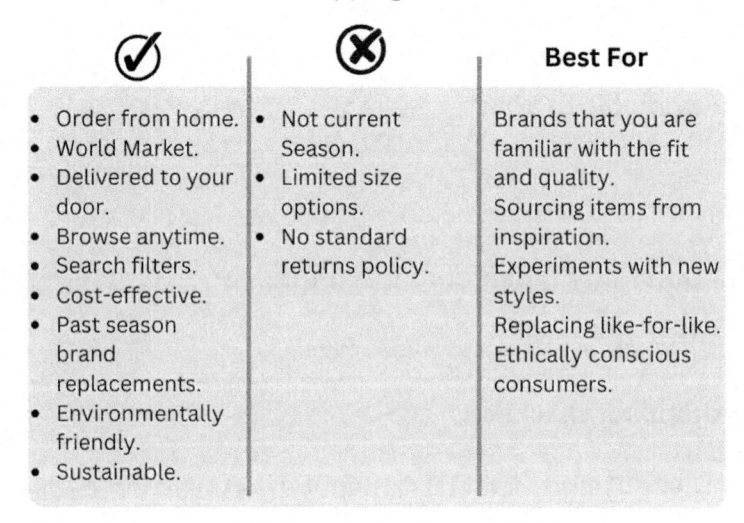

✓	✗	Best For
- Order from home. - World Market. - Delivered to your door. - Browse anytime. - Search filters. - Cost-effective. - Past season brand replacements. - Environmentally friendly. - Sustainable.	- Not current Season. - Limited size options. - No standard returns policy.	Brands that you are familiar with the fit and quality. Sourcing items from inspiration. Experiments with new styles. Replacing like-for-like. Ethically conscious consumers.

Shopping Options Pros & Cons

In-Store Shopping NEW

✓	✗	Best For
• Day out. • Break from screens. • Try on for fit and cut. • Try before you buy online. • Compare sizes. • Compare different cuts and styles. • Feel the fabric. • Use in-store Personal Stylists.	• Added travel time. • Only accessible during shop opening hours.	Trying on new styles. Investment pieces. Brands you know you love. Shopping with friends.

In-Store Shopping PRE-LOVED

✓	✗	Best For
• Day out • Break from screens. • Try on for fit and cut. • Try before you buy online. • Feel the fabric. • Creative finds from all eras. • Low price quality items. • Environmentally friendly. • Sustainable. • Support Charities.	• Added travel time. • Only shop when stores are open. • Limitations with sizing.	Garments from all eras. Trying on new styles. Shopping with friends. Varied choices and types of stores: Charity, Thrift, Op-shops, Vintage Stores, Dress Agencies.

Shopping Options Pros & Cons

In-Store Discount Outlets

✓	✗	Best For
- 60% off designer brands. - Day out. - Break from screens. - Try on for fit and cut. - Feel the fabric.	- End of season or previous season. - Not every size is available. - Items sell quickly so need to buy when seen. - Repeat stock unknown.	High-end brands at discounted prices. Stores include TK.MAXX. Outlets include Oxford -Bicester Village, and Hampshire - Gunwharf Quays

High-End ✓	Low-Cost ✗	When Best For High-End or Low-Cost
- High standard of garment make. - High-quality fabrics. - More details and design features. - Luxury items. - Likely to hold re-sell value. - Become Heirloom pieces. - More likely to be environmentally friendly.	- Decision made on price over style. - Difficult to sell pre-loved therefore likely to end in landfill. - More likely to wear just once. - Production methods often bad for the environment. - Can look cheap.	A High-end is best for: Investment items, statement pieces, coats, footwear and wardrobe upgrades. If you are on a tight budget pre-loved is a great option. Low-cost fast-fashion is cheap, feels & looks cheap. Check out mid priced and choose well.

Shopping Options Pros & Cons

Swishes & Swaps

✓	✗	Best For
• Free clothing. • Good fun. • Linked to Charity fundraising. • Circular fashion. • Environmentally friendly.	• Can be tempting to grab items that are not perfect.	When you have experimental items on your purposeful shopping list. Great for Community collaborations. Easy way to move your surplus on.

Quality	Quantity	When Best For Quality or Quantity
✓ • Last longer. • Heirloom pieces. • Made well. • Luxury fabrics. • Cared for items. • More detailed. • Stylish. ✗ • Some fabrics may require dry cleaning only.	✗ • Take up storage space. • More clothes management time. • Not such precious items. ✓ • More storage space. • More clothes management time. • Not such precious items.	Quality items will form your UPS. They will form a solid level 3 and then easy to style up or down a level, as well as day to night. Quantity is best for uniforms and functional layers. (Think what type of items are sold in packs.)

8. Finishing Touches

When you make a new purchase like a car or a home, it is sold as the standard model, before you choose your finishing options. Further upgrades are available at an additional price; however, if you purchase the test car or show home, you get all the extras which have already been installed whether you would have chosen or needed them. What is the best option for you:

1. The classic standard?
2. A little personalisation?
3. A luxury upgrade?

4. Everything that is on offer?

The finishing touches to your style can be thought of in much the same manner.

1. The basics will give you a natural or classic finish to your style.
2. Add some personalised detail to showcase your UPS.
3. Add your upgrade to develop your Signature Look.
4. Your look will become confused if you choose everything on offer, regardless of UPS or need.

It is consistency that makes your finishing touches authentic and stylish. The finishing touches can make the difference between looking sloppy or stylish. If you love to make a statement, and that is your taste, be consistent and confident in your choices, and they will be a true extension of you. If you are classic, be clear with your finish; it doesn't need to be fussy.

Just as Monet said about his painting,

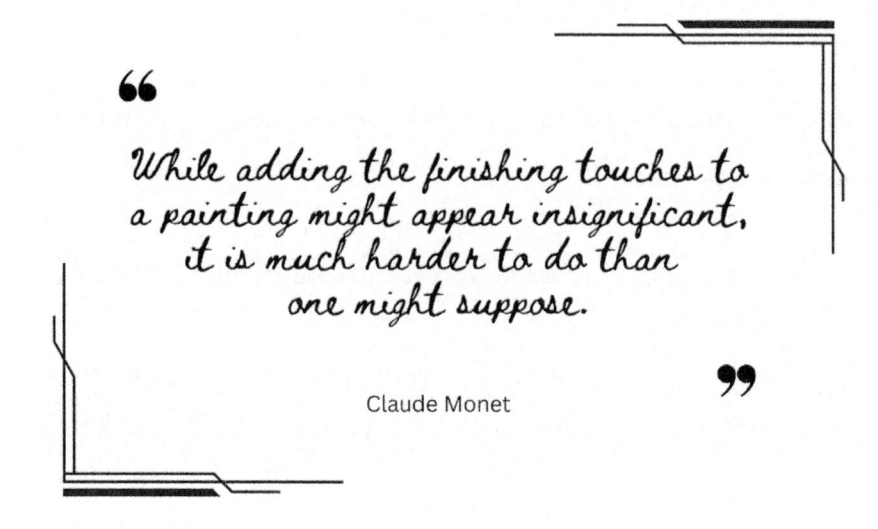

> *While adding the finishing touches to a painting might appear insignificant, it is much harder to do than one might suppose.*
>
> Claude Monet

Consider the finishing touches to your look as a significant part of your overall style.

We are now going to look at how to do this.

8.1 Accessories

I have included accessories in the 'Finishing Touches' chapter for ease of reference. Footwear, bags, belts, scarves, hats, and jewellery all form part of your outfit rather than the finishing touches, but you won't need them all in the same outfit. Hence, it's easier to classify them as accessories for the purposes of this book.

I said it way back in Chapter 2.2 Garments vs. Outfits: Even a one-and-done jumpsuit needs shoes.

Accessories can be used to define and refine your UPS and/or Signature Look. You will have already discovered that your current accessories are the key to maximising outfits because they add style elements, which are what switch the same garment between different Levels of Dress Code, Seasons, and Occasions.

Let's delve deeper into what each accessory does for your style.

Jewellery including brooches, scarves, and belts are timeless and can last a lifetime. They can be used to maintain your UPS when introducing new garments, evolve your style to align with body shape and lifestyle changes, as well as form a signature look if desired.

Footwear, bags, and hats will need updating, but not as often as clothing items. Hats can be used as your UPS but are difficult to pull off as a Signature Look unless you are royalty, like our late Queen Elizabeth II, or a pop star like Jay Kay, the lead singer from the 90s band Jamiroquai.

Footwear and Bags

I've grouped these two together because they are not optional extras; they are part of daily outfits. Both need to be functional, but that certainly does not mean they are unstylish. There are lots of examples of footwear with finished outfits featured through the imagery in the book. Scan the QR code and check the images in Chapter 6.2

A footwear guide can be found on my free downloads page too (if it's not there, it will be because I'm evolving it. You can pop your details in the subscription form and it will be sent to your inbox.)

Scan the QR code to be taken to the Real Women Outfit Library

The bulk of your footwear should be an investment, with attention to fit, comfort, style and longevity. To invest wisely, avoid jumping on a new trend until it's been around for over a year to ensure it's not a fad.

When a footwear style becomes a trend, you can be sure you'll find the style in a comfortable fit lasting 4-5 years. My advice is never to compromise on footwear, no matter how much you think you are saving, because if footwear is uncomfortable, it will cost money to sit in a shoebox. For comfortable, stylish shoes, choose from shoemaker brands rather than clothes brands that favour fashion over comfort.

Russell & Bromley, Jones the Bootmaker, Moda in Pelle, Clarks, and Birkenstocks will all look after your feet better than picking up a non-branded shoe from a fast fashion store.

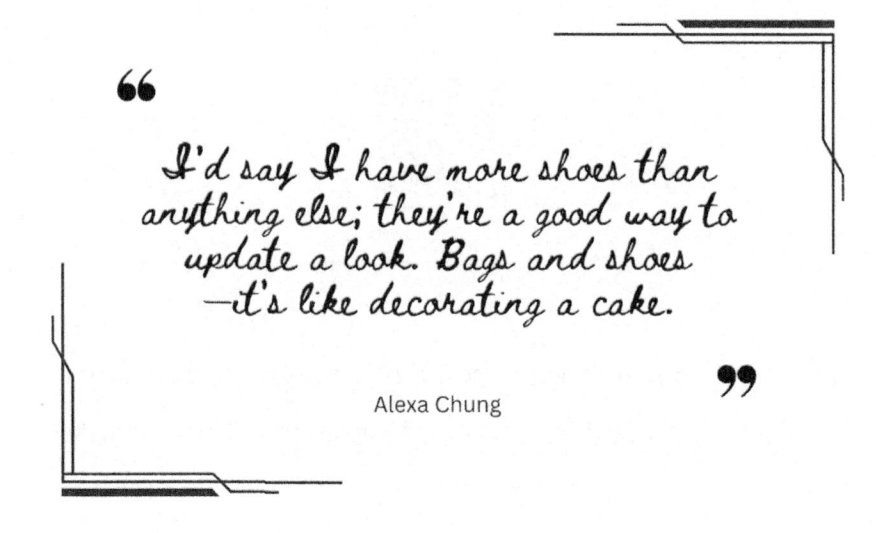

> *I'd say I have more shoes than anything else; they're a good way to update a look. Bags and shoes —it's like decorating a cake.*
>
> Alexa Chung

Bags come in three general sizes: small handbag or clutch for your essentials like keys, phone, money, and a compact; medium day bag for your essentials plus larger items such as sunglasses, umbrella, foldaway tote, hairbrush, and makeup; and large work bag or tote for laptops, books, extra layers, etc.

Your UPS will determine if your bag is a statement, the focal point of your outfit, or a subtle extension. As with shoes, bags are generally an investment; however, seasonal bags like beach bags and shopping totes are likely to be replaced more often.

Bags are also big business amongst the wealthy and collectors. If you like your designer labels, check out the pre-loved market. If you are looking to invest, it has been said that bags increase in value more than gold. Handbag expert and authentication manager at The Luxury Closet said,

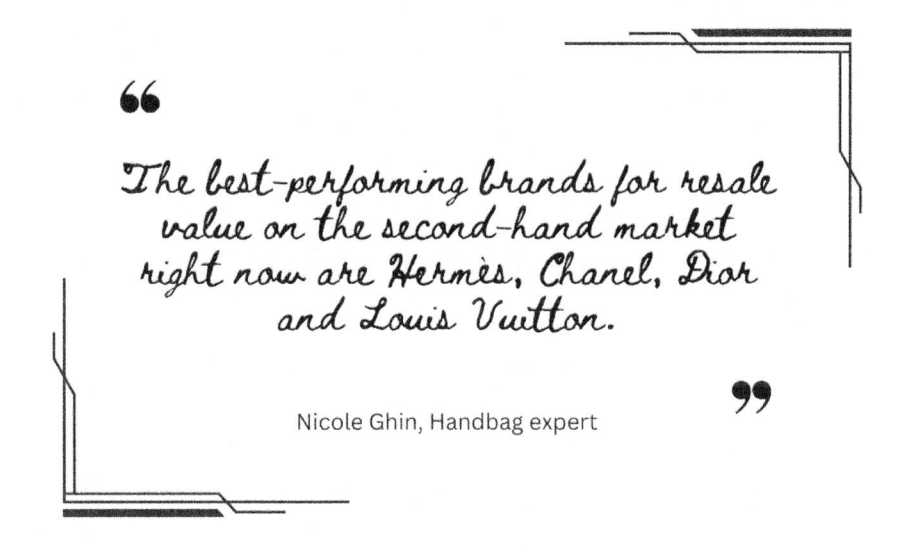

> "The best-performing brands for resale value on the second-hand market right now are Hermès, Chanel, Dior and Louis Vuitton.
>
> Nicole Ghin, Handbag expert

If you are not a fan of leather or your ethics don't care for leather, choose textured fabrics and embossed plastic. Many materials, such as ring pulls, ocean plastics, and even sweet wrappers, can be creatively used to make a good bag.

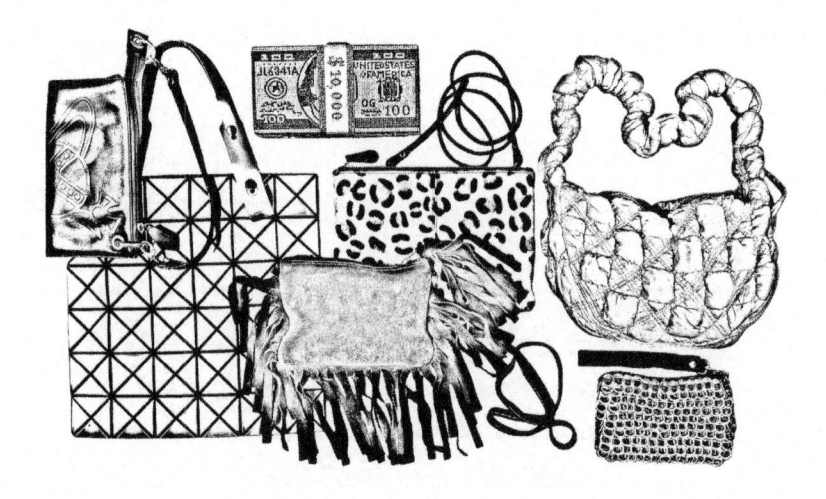

Here are a few fun bags - all are functional

Unusual bags and bags with a story from the designer make great talking points, like a piece of art. When used as the focal point of your look, they can direct attention away from aspects of your outfit. So, if you are feeling like a 'cover-up' day, select an outfit with minimal detail, such as a one-and-done dress or jumpsuit, and add a statement bag.

Pairing bags and shoes, and taking a photograph of your pairings, will save oodles of time in the long run. The number of times I hear women say they have forgotten about a bag or shoes, I know pairing them up in advance is time well spent. If like me, you keep shoes in their boxes and bags in their dust bags it is impossible to see what you have otherwise.

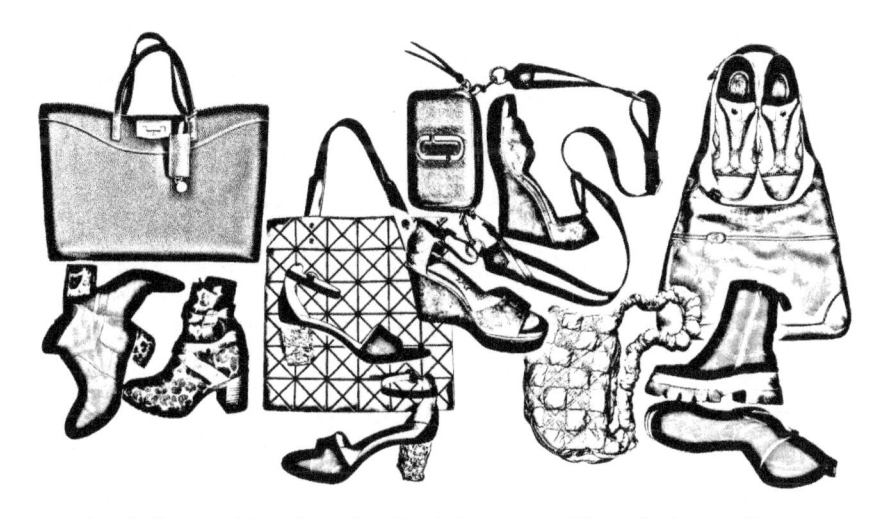

Bags & Shoes work together as functional pieces you can't leave the house without. Pair them together in advance for easy finishing touches to any Outfit.

Hats & Scarves

Winter warmers or part of an outfit? To remain true to your UPS, hats and scarves should not be a matching set. Leave that look to children.

A silk scarf is an all-year-round accessory that can be styled to add interest to any outfit, a one-and-done dress or jumpsuit, and add pattern to a plain outfit, or vice versa. There are endless ways to tie a scarf and that's just around the neck. They can be tied to a handbag, or worn as a head scarf, but my favourite is the larger square-shaped ones that can be tied into bolero-style cover-ups that won't fall off your shoulders. More details on scarf tying and styling are available – drop me a line if you'd like to know more.

Winter warmer scarves are seasonal - but not limited to the winter season. A chunky knit or oversized woollen scarf can be quite the statement piece that works over a jumper dress, knitted cardi-coat, or a mid-season jacket. Remember Sally's story in Chapter 7.2, Finding Style Inspiration.

Hat-wearing is all about what's happening with your hair. If you've styled your hair around your headpiece, what happens when you take the hat off, or will you need to keep the hat on until you have a mirror and hairbrush to hand?

Regular hat wearers have the hair for a hat. Occasional hat wearers do so for specific reasons, like sun protection, sports peaks, race day wear, or wedding attire. There is also a category of non-hat wearers. They are not for everyone.

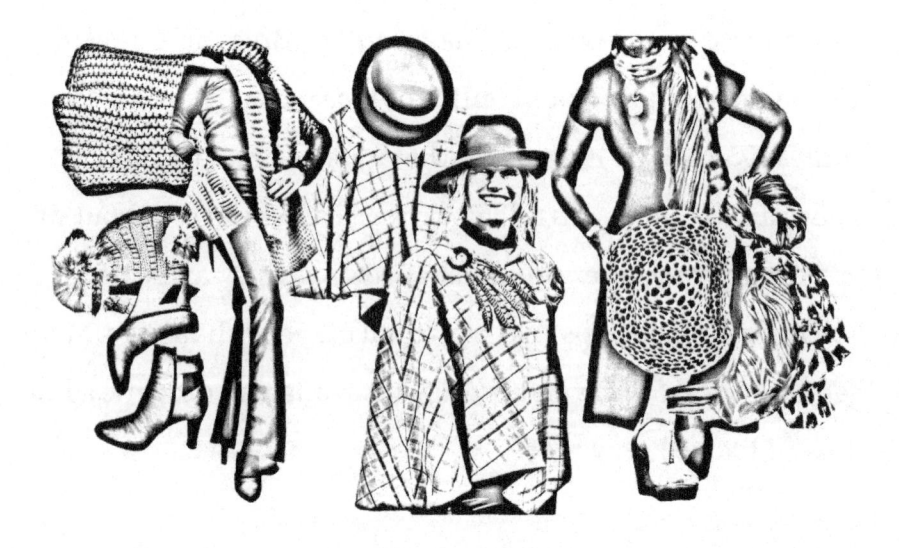

Hats & Scarves are like shoes & bags. They work harmoniously to complete a look, even when added as the statement piece.

Belts & Jewellery

Belts are like jewellery, adding personalised detail and the finishing touches to an overall outfit. They can be as subtle as a soft tie in the fabric to add shape and secure the clothing to the body or act as a fastening to tie a garment closed. The other end of the spectrum is a rigid wide belt in a contrasting colour with a large or specific decorative buckle.

The jewellery spectrum also ranges from practical to highly decorative. For example, a plain wedding band declares your marital status with no particular stylisation, and a wristwatch keeps time, yet rings and watches can also be statement pieces that contribute to your UPS. Jewellery items extend to brooches, pins, body piercings, and tiaras.

Belts and jewellery can extend an outfit by linking colours or textures, or, like bags or footwear, they can be the focal point, statement, or signature piece of an outfit. One of the Chapter 7.1 images shows an example of signature look jewellery.

Glasses

Both the spectacle kind and sun shades. If you wear glasses

regularly with many different outfits, it is essential to select frames that compliment your face shape and features or create a conscious statement. You may need more than one pair to work with your UPS on every level of dress code. If you wear frames full-time, they are more than an accessory; they are the ultimate extension of you and your signature look, whether you want them to be or not.

There are formulas that match face shape to the best frame shape, which is a good starting point however, the reflection you see in a full-length mirror will tell you more.

I did mean to say 'full-length' mirror, because you are not just a head, and your frames need to suit your face and the rest of you.

The late Iris Apfel, featured in Chapter 1.3 - Age & Dressing, and Anna Wintour mentioned in Chapter 7.1 - Signature Looks, are both known for their signature look frames yet both have completely different UPSs.

Accessories - Summary

- Accessories are part of your curated outfit, essential to your UPS, and instrumental in differentiation between

levels of dress code.
- Over time, if you discover a particular accessory you love and curate with every outfit, it can become your signature look.
- Daily footwear and bags are investment pieces, with additional season and reason pieces as and when necessary.
- Jewellery, scarves and belts can be timeless, make perfect heirloom pieces, and create effortless stylish detail when antique, vintage or retro mixed with new.

Suggested Actions

1. Do not choose an accessory solely for function. Like clothing, there are enough options and technical advances for function and style to co-exist.
2. Re-assess your accessories audit, pairing bags and shoes that can be worn together, and adding scarves or hats if you wear them.
3. Add any missing accessories that complement your UPS to your purposeful shopping list.
4. For accessory shopping follow the same process as for clothing but check out new designers on Etsy or plan to visit Vintage fayres and look up charities such as BottleTops.
5. Accessories are a great way to progress your USP and keep it evolving.

Take photographs of your bag and shoe pairings as you go –

you can have more than one set of footwear with each bag, and vice versa. Keep a printout of your photographs in your wardrobe.

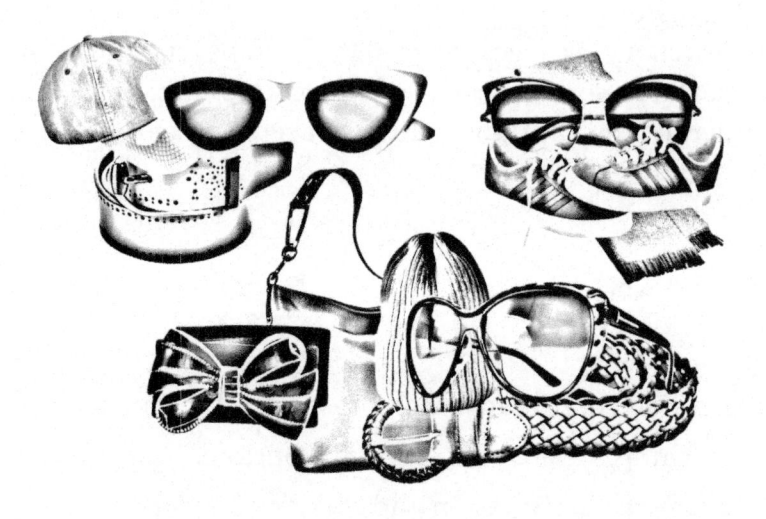

Edit your Accessories like outfits.
Not to wear all at once, just ready to style the finishing touches on outfits across seasons and to level UP and DOWN.

8.2 Skin, Hair & Make-up

This is basically personal grooming, hygiene and caring for your skin, hair, nails and teeth. No one finds chapped lips, chipped nail polish, body odour, bad breath or hair sprouting from anywhere except your head attractive or stylish. Spend a minimum of 15 minutes daily on personal grooming and check your fully groomed status in a full-length mirror.

In addition to your daily grooming, there is the option of makeup, which, if applied, is part of your UPS. Your makeup application will also evolve to align with your lifestyle and can be used as a style element to switch between levels or a consistent feature throughout levels as a signature look.

Make-Up

Whether you are a seasoned makeup wearer or not, a little

enhancement to your natural assets shows you care and keeps you looking fresh. What doesn't look fresh is applying the same full-face makeup look for decades.

My advice on make-up is to think about these four items as the basics:

1. Brow pencil
2. Mascara
3. Blusher
4. Lipstick or lip balm

These four basics all work by adding lost definition to the areas of your face that fade with age. Touching up your eyebrow hair and eyelashes will frame your eyes, blush or bronzer adds colour to your cheeks or contours your face shape, and lipstick or balm can be clear, glossy, or coloured to your taste to keep your lips protected and visible.

Beyond these four basics, for further advice, ask the people in your life that you think manage their make-up well or book an appointment with a make-up consultant. All department stores that sell make-up have trained make-up artists who specialise in skin care along with the products they are selling. Take along images of make-up looks you like; this can be done on Pinterest, or you may already have an idea from earlier inspiration and tell the consultant what you want to achieve. For example, you might want to achieve a daily routine that takes less than 10 minutes with a lesson on how to apply makeup or specifics such as how to cover skin blemishes, create an even skin tone, conceal under-eye bags, apply contouring technique, choose a lip colour or gloss that is suitable for daily wear, or how to create an evening smoky-eye without going OTT on black pencil and accidentally looking like 80's goth Siouxsie Sioux!

If you are new to makeup or you realise your application hasn't evolved in the last decade, YouTube is another great educator. Search video tutorials by date, for example, 'make-up tutorial 2024', for the latest looks, application techniques, and products.

If you are a regular makeup user, semi-permanent makeup, micro-blading, and an array of high-definition lash and brow treatments are now commonplace. Ask to see before-and-after pictures and testimonials to ensure you like the practitioner's style.

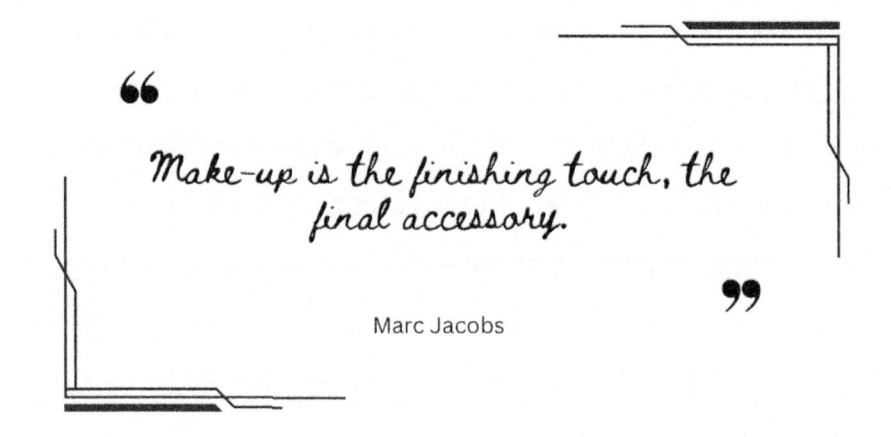

> *Make-up is the finishing touch, the final accessory.*
>
> — Marc Jacobs

Skincare

Skincare is a specialist topic in your grooming and hygiene routine. In some cases, expert intervention is necessary. There are so many products on the market, all claiming to do different things, so my advice here is similar to my makeup advice and starts with three basics: cleanser, moisturiser, and sun protection.

If you feel your skincare routine needs a refresh, ask someone you know who has good skin; otherwise, book in with a beauty consultant or skin clinic for a consultation. Most are free of charge or offset the consultation fee against products you go ahead and purchase thereafter. Be aware of unnecessary upsells and always ask why a product is good and what it does for your skin.

I'm not a fan of skin toner or 'wash off' moisturisers, and I love gradual tanning lotions. You are as individual as our UPS when it comes to skincare, so do your research, take advantage of tester sample sachets, and refresh your routine as your skin and lifestyle change.

My final word on skin is about your legs. We tend to focus on our face and neck skin; however, many of my clients worry about exposing bare legs, even if just from below the knee. Do you regularly exfoliate and moisturise your legs? Both actions massage your legs, which supports circulation and helps break down fat deposits beneath the skin's surface to create a smoother skin tone. If you are pale-skinned like me, using a moisturiser with a tanning agent to massage after exfoliating means smoother, tanned legs ready for skirts, dresses, and wide-leg cropped trousers. Do remember to wear a tanning mitt, or you'll end up with orangey-brown palms!

> **"Glowing skin is always in."**

Hair Care

We are not all born with a mop of thick, silky hair with a perfect hairline, and if you are, there is no guarantee your luscious locks will last a lifetime. Instead, characteristics such as fine, wispy, frizzy, dry or lank, and lacking body or volume are more associated with describing the average hair type. As a person ages, their hair changes, not all in the same way or at the same rate, because our hair follicles are unique structures. Add in illness, disease, and medication, which affect hair structure and condition, and we have a topic that is too big to list every hairstyle and who they suit.

The basic principles are to know your hair's limitations but not to keep one style forever. Consider a tweak if you have been sporting the same hairstyle for a few decades. So far, you have been asking your stylist to add more colour or products to counter the change as much as possible or letting the same cut organically change as your hair changes. Consider an active, defined change and ask your stylist for their thoughts. It could be hair parting position, adding a fringe, colour, length, layers, curl, straightening, style of blow dry, or testing a new finishing product. Let your hair stylist know you are conscious of looking dated as you've had the same cut for a while and ask them what options would work on your hair type. If you don't have a regular hairstylist, start now. Next time you have your hair cut, book your next appointment by asking for the same stylist because you would like advice and suggestions about what options would work well for your hair type.

If you decide to make more significant changes to your hairstyle, be patient because it takes a little while to get used to a new style. Ask friends what they think, permitting them to be truthful, but be aware – your nearest and dearest are unlikely to be prepared for change, and if so, they will say, "I liked you just how you were; why are you bothering?". That is about them, and they haven't answered your question.

Or when someone you trust tells you they don't like it, ask them why. They might say, "Because it's not you". If that is the response, it indicates that it's not that they don't like it; they're just not prepared for change.

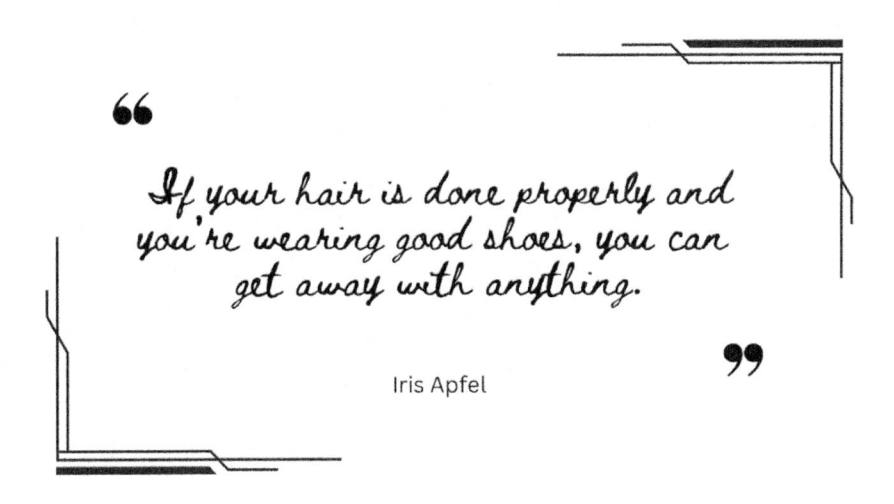

> *If your hair is done properly and you're wearing good shoes, you can get away with anything.*
>
> Iris Apfel

Injectables & Extras

Let's make it very clear—injectables and extras are not required to be awesomely stylish. They are a fast-growing market based around avoiding the signs of ageing skin, developing so rapidly that it is not likely to disappear any time soon. It is worth mentioning, if only to reassure you, that when you see a 60-year-old looking 35, they are most likely using some form of age-defying treatment.

At the time of writing, these treatments are part of an unregulated industry in the UK, which pushes the responsibility onto us to do adequate research and checks and consult the necessary experts before injecting toxins or piercing our skin.

I am familiar with the following treatments because I have clients who work in the industry and clients who have experienced the procedures. I've combined words from both sets of clients to form a very brief description of some treatments and their intended results.

Starting with Botulinum toxin aka Botox

It's an injection that works by freezing muscles to stop the movement of the surface skin. Commonly used around the forehead, brow, and eyes to prevent skin wrinkles such as crows-feet and forehead lines. Freezing the muscle also freezes facial expression, so it's not a secret anti-ageing treatment because a frozen forehead is detectable. Botox injections are also used to control the symptoms of severe underarm sweating. A welcome cure for sufferers of this condition.

Radio Frequency Microneedling or RFM

RFM is an aesthetic procedure that uses tiny needles and radio-frequency waves to rejuvenate the skin by utilising a form of controlled skin injury. The procedure leads to a tightening effect, improving fine lines, wrinkles, loose crêpe skin, and overall skin tone. In 2021, Judy Murray, the mum of famous tennis star Sir Andy Murray, underwent the treatment, which reportedly took 10 years off her looks. It is also effective in treating acne scars and stretch marks.

Unlike previous procedures, **dermal fillers** are injections of filler substances that instantly plump out wrinkles and smooth lines, producing results immediately.

None of these procedures last a lifetime and are typically

repeated, costing well into the hundreds.

Skin, Hair And Makeup - Summary

- Hygiene and grooming are essential to the finishing touches of how you present your style.
- Cosmetics, including hair treatments and makeup, are a personal preference, and cosmetic procedures such as injectables are non-essential to your overall style and are purely down to individual choice.
- Trends in cosmetic looks constantly change in the same way as clothing.
- If you fail to evolve your cosmetic habits to align with your lifestyle, your look will become dated and unstylish.
- This doesn't mean you have to embark on a cosmetic regime if you don't want to, it simply means if you are big into cosmetics remember not to get stuck in a dated habit because things do change.

The history of hair dying, for example, used to be considered so shameful, that ladies were hidden behind curtains in salons so as not to be seen indulging in anti-ageing procedures. At that time, chemicals were too dangerous to DIY at home. By the mid-1950s, chemical advances and the "Does She or Doesn't She?" Clairol campaign put hair dying on the map. Now an estimated 66% of women dye their hair to cover up grey.

In recent years, non-essential shops including hair salons closed for some time during the World Covid-19 pandemic and as a result, there was an increase in the embracing of greying hair. The trend that followed was the 'pre-grey hair generation' dying their hair silver-grey and platinum-grey to deliberately look grey!

Suggested Actions

If you have had the same skincare or make-up routine for over a decade or feel ready for a refreshed look, book time out in your diary to:

1. Watch YouTube tutorials by searching by date, application technique and latest products. Look for 'sponsored' videos for discounts on products you wish to buy, or make a note of what they are and check them out in a retail store asking for samples.
2. Book a consultation or facial with a skin expert, making it clear you are looking for a daily routine and suitable products for your skin type.
3. Check out your local make-up retailers and book a session and lesson with a make-up artist, making it clear you are seeking a fresh look that you can apply yourself. Arrive wearing your usual make-up and

discuss what they intend to do to freshen up your look before you remove your makeup.

If you have had the same hairstyle for over a decade or feel ready for a fresh look, collect some images or make a Pinterest board to show ideas to your hairdresser. Ask the advice of your hairdresser too. They will know what styles are new and what is possible with your hair type and budget.

Extra Info

If you are considering cosmetic procedures in the UK, "The current regulatory framework places few restrictions on who can perform non-surgical cosmetic procedures. The government recognises the concerns about the lack of regulation in this field and the potential dangers that this poses to the public."

https://www.gov.uk/government/consultations/licensing-of-non-surgical-cosmetic-procedures/the-licensing-of-non-surgical-cosmetic-procedures-in-england

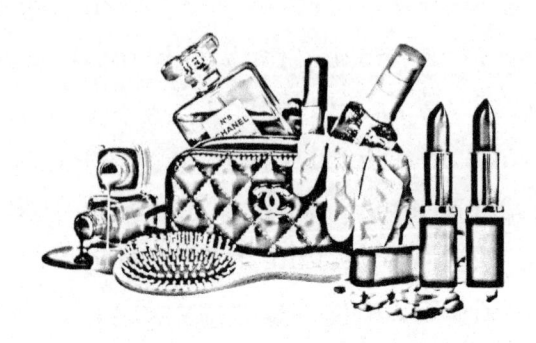

9. The Wardrobe Evolution Cycle

If you kept every item you encountered throughout adulthood, successfully managing your clothes and remaining stylish for a lifetime would be near impossible.

The chapters in this book have taken you through a cycle that teaches what clothes you need at any given time, how to curate them into outfits, how to figure out your UPS, how to align your clothes with your lifestyle, and how to refresh your clothes while identifying when it's time to move older clothes on. It works in a cycle that can be continually repeated; however, we went into it in more depth, diving into explanations about the stages and how to do them for the first time.

If you continue the cycle forever, it will become second nature, and your wardrobe will never contain items that don't serve you or your current lifestyle. Instead, your wardrobe will evolve into a flow of managed stylish outfits that are your 2nd SKIN. An inner closet that lifts your mood and brings you joy, and an outer armour that will give you confidence to face your day ahead.

The Wardrobe Evolution Cycle

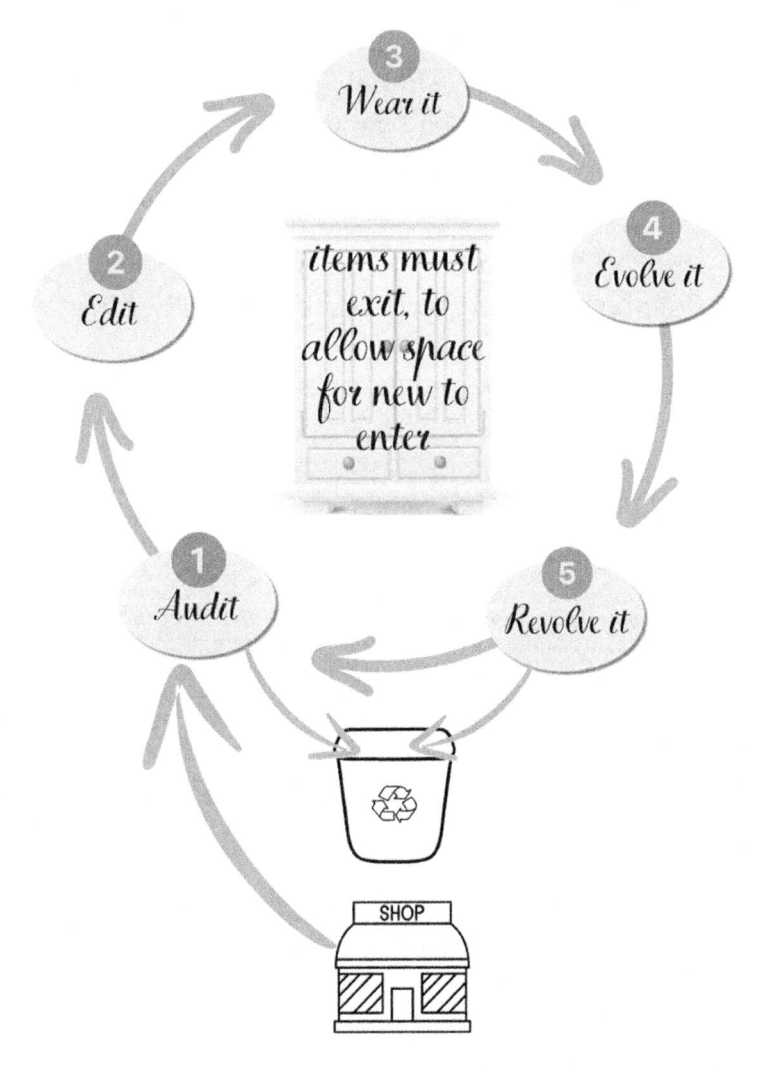

1. Audit
2. Edit
3. Wear it
4. Evolve it
5. Revolve it

items must exit, to allow space for new to enter

The Wardrobe Evolution Cycle - Summary

Here are the stages of The Wardrobe Evolution Cycle, which are the 5 Steps:

1. **Audit** – Never put a garment back in your wardrobe that is not 10 out of 10 today, including repairs or alteration. Chapter 5, Wardrobe Therapy Part 1-The Audit.

2. **Edit** – Every item must be paired with other pieces to form a bank of ready-to-wear outfit combinations. Chapter 6, Wardrobe Therapy Part 2 -The Edit.

3. **Wear-it** – Check your outfits align with your current lifestyle on every level, making you feel and look your best. Chapter 4, Daily Dress Codes. Chapter 6, Maximising your Clothes.

4. **Evolve-it** – Tweak, refine and define what you feel, wear and see. Chapter 7, Evolving Your UPS. Chapter 8, Finishing Touches.

5. **Revolve-it** – When your outfit no longer feels 10 out of 10 move the items out and refresh by bringing new ones in. Chapter 5, Wardrobe Therapy Part 1 & Chapter 7. Evolving Your UPS.

Suggested Actions

If you get stuck at any of the 5 Steps, at any time on your lifelong journey of personal style discovery, my suggested action is to revisit Chapters 1 and 2, YOU Laid Bare and

CLOTHES Unpicked.

The complexities of body image, the obstacles of self-esteem, and the passage of time can so easily interrupt the flow of your style and the transformative power of your clothing.

Then, use the references in Chapter 3, STYLE Formulas, to choose your best confidence booster. Take the action and then step straight back on The Wardrobe Evolution Cycle.

The Wardrobe Evolution Cycle

1. Audit	2. Edit	3. Wear it	4. Evolve it	5. Revolve it
Do you: • Love it? • 100% Fit? • Condition?	Flat-lay Outfits Ideas Make a shopping list	Wear your Outfits Level UP & Level DOWN	Style across Seasons Progress your UPS	• Replace/Buy • Up-Fashion • Donate/Sell/Recycle

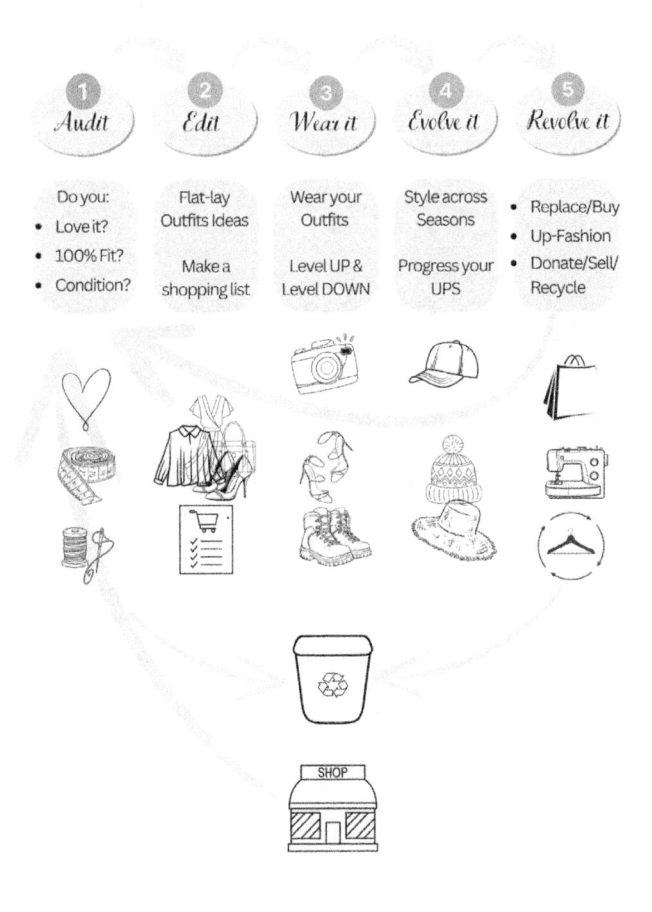

10. Not The End

---•---

Most journeys start at the beginning and finish at the end. But not a wardrobe of clothes. Your collection started way before you picked up this book, and it won't end now that you have reached the final chapter. Your wardrobe evolves with life, and that's exactly what 2nd SKIN conveys.

The Wardrobe Evolution Cycle is a method I have been using to manage my own wardrobe and client's wardrobes for over three decades. I don't teach it to clients; I do it for them, returning when needed, auditing, editing, maximising, increasing their confidence, and bringing them instant joy when they open their wardrobe door.

I have taught you the secrets to my method in this book. These teachings allude to continually evolving your clothes collection. You already automatically revolve your collection by taking items out of your wardrobe to get dressed and replacing them afterwards while adding and losing pieces as you go.

Evolving your clothes means turning off your automation to consciously assess whether your items are serving you well and having the confidence to seek better if they're not. Never make do, never settle for second best, and never give up.

There will be times in your life when change is obvious, which happens quickly and relatively fuss-free, periods of plateau with minimal change, and difficult times, which are often when change is unwelcome. Life's changes still require you to get dressed, and with the right mindset, your second skin, aka clothes, has the power to enhance every stage.

Dressing well, loving your wardrobe, and using what you wear to feel great, look good, and perform your best starts with believing you can. It is possible. And it is possible for a lifetime. No explanations, excuses, blaming your body, saying you didn't have time or you couldn't afford it, and no saying you don't care.

Do care and be proud.

If you think clothes aren't your thing… Sorry? Clothes are everybody's thing; getting dressed is a legal requirement (!), so embrace, explore and enjoy it while you can!

If you don't love your body, then choose clothes. Love and feel the power of being beautiful in your 2nd SKIN.

"There is no best-before or sell-by date on being stylish."

Thank you for reading,

love Sarah

Pssst. Wear next?

(pun intended!)

Online Courses, including Clothing Fit & Fabric, Garment Alterations for both sewists and non-sewists.

The Stylish Wardrobe Club – free private FB group.

Oh, and did I mention book No.2? "Clothes Foraging" is coming next.

The continuation of the Digital Outfit Library of Real Women.

Visit www.myvos.co.uk

Glossary

In writing 2nd SKIN I've used words and terms familiar to clothes-obsessed individuals yet may not be as familiar to you. I also noticed some words used to describe clothing style describe other things too.

So here are the meanings in this book:

A
Alterations – *The process of changing, modifying or adjusting the fit, style, or look of garments, for the better.*

B

Bias Cut – A method of garment construction that uses the diagonal cross-grain of a fabric, referred to as cut-on-the-bias, to create garment shapes that skim body curves.

Bolero Style – Jackets or cardigans that are shorter in length finishing higher than the waistline.

Boyfriend Jeans – A casual, oversized pair of jeans, that are usually rolled up at the ankles and create a laid-back look - as if you've just nabbed them from your boyfriend's wardrobe.

Brand – A business or label that operates within the fashion industry creating a reputation that causes people to buy into their style, ethics and values.

C

Capsule Wardrobe – Also referred to as Capsule Collection is a limited number of items that mix and match with each other to make a multitude of outfit options.

Colour Analysis - A formula that tests different shades of colour against a person's skin tone, eye colour and hair colour to identify which clothing colours would suit the person the best.

Curated Outfit – The completed outcome of individual garments and items that are put together to create the end outfit, including footwear, outerwear and accessories.

Cut – The cut of a garment refers to the shape of the item. However, fabric type has a bearing on the cut; therefore, cut and fit can be confused because an identical cut in a different fabric type can sit on the body differently causing the fit and look to be different too.

D

Décolletage – *A woman's neck and chest area as revealed by a lower-cut garment neckline.*

Denim – *Traditionally a firm, durable, cotton twill fabric, woven with indigo and white threads that create a dark blue fabric on the outside, and white frayed threads when torn, distressed, or left as a raw edge.*

Drape – *A floppy, fluid fabric that hangs close to the body and swishes away from the body line when in motion.*

Dress Code - *Outfits in your UPS approproiate for what where you are and what you are doing.*

F

Fabric – *Any material that clothes are made from, including wovens, knits, leathers and plastics.*

Fad – *A style, look, or garment that is short-lived, typically seen for just one season or reason.*

Fashion – *The marketing and selling of clothes.*

Flat Lay – *Also referred to as flat-styling or flat-lay-style; is the method of laying clothes and accessories out on a flat surface in position of wear, to get an idea of how they would look like as an outfit.*

French Tuck - *Wearing a top where a section of the front is tucked into a waistband, but the back is left loose and untucked. Also known as the half-tuck or one-hand tuck.*

F-Row – *The front row seats of a runway show.*

G

Garment – *An item of clothing, which can be referred to as simply a 'piece'.*

H

Heirloom – *Clothing items that can be passed down through generations. Often classic or iconic pieces that can be styled with current looks.*

I

Indigo – *Indigo is the blue dye that gives blue jeans their colour. It is unique because it gathers around the core of the fabric fibres rather than infiltrating the centre. This is why denim fades over time as each washing cycle removes indigo from the fabric.*

Inspo – *Abbreviation of inspiration.*

J

Jersey – *A fabric that is defined by its knitted, looped-together construction, making it a stretchy fabric rather than a stable woven material.*

K

Knit – *Garment fabric made by interlocking loops with knitting needles or by machine.*

L

Level Dressing - *Categorising clothes into 5-levels in allignment with lifestyle activities.*

Loungewear – *Comfortable clothing that you wear at home, but not necessarily to bed.*

LYCRA® - *The trademarked brand name of synthetic elastic fibres known as elastane (spandex in the U.S.) which is the element that makes a fabric stretch and spring back to its intended shape.*

M

Material – *In the context of style is the fabric clothes are made from.*

O

One-And-Done – *Dresses and jumpsuits which are one item of clothing that covers both top and bottom.*

Outfit Combo – *The combination of individual garments and pieces used to create an entire finished, ready-to-wear outfit.*

Outfit Selfie – *A snap of yourself wearing a finished outfit combo.*

P

Pre-loved – *Items that have already been purchased brand new and are now being re-sold, previously referred to as second-hand. Even if an item has never been worn and is in its original packaging with tags, it is still considered pre-loved. An item can be sold endless times.*

R

Re-Cycled – *Garments that have been re-styled, re-made, or repurposed to keep the garment or garment fabric in circulation rather than discarded.*

Re-Fashion – *Upgrade or fix a garment to make it different and still wearable, also referred to as Up-fashion.*

S

Separates - *Individual items of clothing, such as skirts, tops,* *jackets, or trousers, suitable for wearing in different combinations.*

Signature Look – *A distinguished look that is instantly recognisable and related to a particular person's style.*

Sustainable Clothing - *Garments production that considers environmental and human impact. It also includes practices like re-selling and pre-loved, which extends the life of clothes keeping them in circulation for longer.*

T

Trend – *A look or style that is developing and becoming more common and lasts for about 5 years.*

U

Up-Fashion – *The same as re-fashion, also referred to as Up-cycle, is to upgrade or fix a garment to make it different and keep it in circulation for longer.*

UPS - *Unique Personal Style.*

W

Wardrobe Audit – *Sort through one's clothes to remove all items that no longer fit or serve a purpose.*

Wardrobe Edit – *Sorting clothing items and accessories into wearable outfits.*

Wardrobe Flow – *An audited, edited collection of clothes that serve a person in all aspects of their daily life, at any given time.*

Resources

Health & Well-being Experts:

Holistic Transformation Therapist
Janie Whittemore - janiewhittemore.com

Body Confidence Activist
Rachel Peru - liberteltd.com

Shiatsu Practitioner & Chinese Medicine Therapist
Andrea Marsh - cotswoldmenopause.co.uk

Psychotherapist and Hypnotherapist
Dipti Tait - diptitait.com

Integrative Health Practitioner & Health Coach
Jessica Green - jessicagreenwellness.com

The Future of Clothing Well-being:

Clothing and the Planet News:

www.earth.org

Sustainable fashion advice:
www.goodonyou.eco

Pre-loved Dress Agencies:
Revamp, Cheltenham Gloucestershire
Encore, Cirencester Gloucestershire

Clothes Donation/Collection sites:
icollectclothes.co.uk, donateclothes.uk, recycle-more.co.uk. werecycleclothes.org, Anglo Doorstep.

Clothes Selling Sites:
Vinted, Depop, FB Marketplace, eBay, Vestiare Collective, Luxe collective, Olio App

IG links:
@erica_davies @carla.rockmore @emmahill @tamumcpherson @iconaccidental @Trinnywoodall @funmiford @seasonsofella @jessontheplussize @thecreativeclassicist @myenglishcountrycottage @stylebynanny

Weekly Style Fix:
Who Wear What, Harper's Bazaar, The Style Times Magazine

Cosmetic Procedure Info, England:
www.gov.uk/government/consultations/licensing-of-non-surgical-cosmetic-procedures/the-licensing-of-non-surgical-cosmetic-procedures-in-england

Acknowledgements

There are many people I owe enormous thanks to for helping me bring project '2nd SKIN', out of my head and into a book. Many of them, not knowing how their contribution of support, words of wisdom and encouragement kept me going; and to the women who allowed me to take photos of them and their clothes – I needed you all and thank you all from my heart.

As promised, I shall not reveal the names of the awesome women who contributed to over 200 photographs. Some of you were unsuspecting and took a little persuasion, some of you let me into your homes for a selection of outfits; and others sent your outfit selfies directly. You know who you are, and I sincerely thank you - My real woman, whose body shapes are gorgeously 'human' and well-dressed. THANK YOU!

To Sara, Paula, Nicky, Debs, Jackie, B, and Carrie. Your patience and honesty have been priceless, and I will be forever grateful for your thoughts and direction that shaped the final book. You might be hearing from me regarding book No.2!

Jessica, Rachel, Janie, Dipti and Andrea, I thank you all for your expert input in matters of the Mind and Body. Confident dressing at it's best, starts on the inside.

The Authors & Co. family, Abi, Carol, Deanne, Shelley, and Lisa. Without 'The One' team, the writing circle, and the camaraderie of others on the course, my book would still be in a drawer.

AnnMarie 'beginabook.com' Reynolds. The superstar I met by chance, who turned my unedited words into a flowable read *and* finally made me feel proud that I've written a book.

A special thanks to Fliss. You've kept me sane, taught me more English in the last 18 months than I dreamt possible, and yuo've been with me from the start, literally at me side, often at a *drop-of-hat* to rescue me from self-doubt. Thank you again, my friend.

My husband, Mr Cross. You've lived and breathed this project with me. You've supported me on every level giving me the freedom, time and space to *get it done*. I thank you, love you, and can't live without you. I hope you like it; I think I'm looking forward to your critique. & my children, who never question what idea mums got next – I hope you like it too. Do you think you'll read it?

About The Author

Personal style runs through Sarah's veins. The youngest of 3 siblings, Sarah was raised in a bustling seaside town on the west coast of England. As a child, she spent hours watching her mum at the sewing machine, making many of her own clothes and re-styling her older sister's hand-me-downs to give them a fresh appeal before they became her clothes. Stepping out in bespoke clothes stayed with Sarah as it became her norm to tweak garments, making them unique or custom-made versions of the latest pieces seen on the runway.

During her study years, Sarah bought any items she could find from thrift shops, with only one criterion - it had to be the highest quality fabric. (OK, maybe 2 criteria – a designer label in it too!) Size, style, colour or shape didn't matter, she had the skill, and the eye to make anything wearable or sellable.

Sarah often reflects on the time she spent at the start of her career as a fashion designer. Three decades ago, fast fashion was in its heyday and Sarah found herself right in the core of the movement, although it never sat comfortably with her. She says, "For someone who loves clothes, I've been exceptionally lucky to have experienced the fashion industry from inside and out; discovering both the good and the bad". She goes on to say, "I went full circle in a short space of time realising that the shift in cheap clothes had flaws on many levels. Half a generation later, I'm teaching Fashion & Clothing to school leavers and adults returning to education alike in a quest to progress *their* careers. Those years gave me another insight into the critical importance the next generations are putting on clothing both personally and commercially."

Sarah continues to help women use the power of clothes to elevate their mood just by opening their Wardrobe door. She is regularly featured on local radio shows and hosts a women's business group. When she's not helping others feel the joy of clothes, Sarah splits her time between retreating to the coast to sail the seas with her husband and enjoying social time with family and friends.

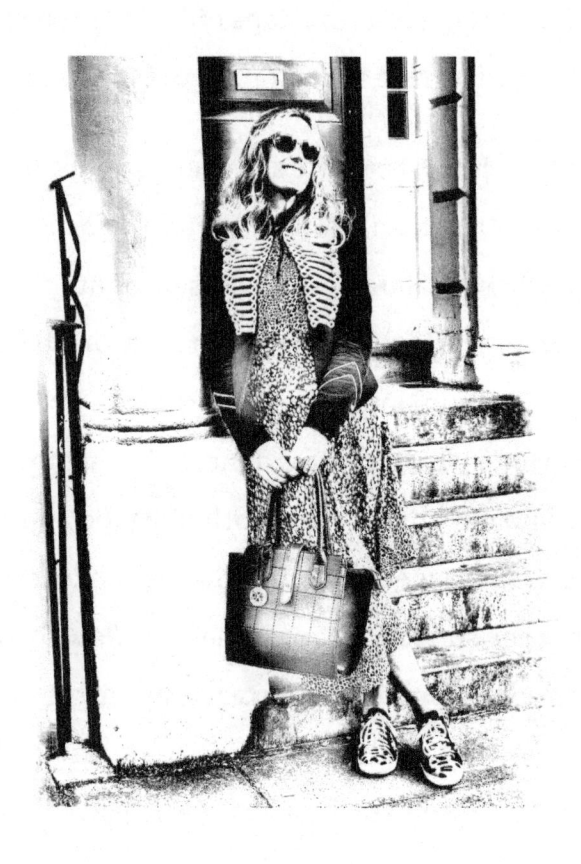

Printed in Great Britain
by Amazon